Navigating the Minefield of Cancer Treatment

Joann Temple Dennett

Cover and Book Design by Sandra Rush

ISBN: 978-1492269601

Printed in the United States of America

This book is dedicated to my husband

Roger

without whom I wouldn't want to have
traveled through this life.

Contents

Contents

Contents

Contents

PREFACE

IN THE BEGINNING

My cancer diagnosis wasn't sudden. It hovered in the background for more than a year after an x-ray before routine knee surgery revealed "suspicious anomalies" of unknown origin in my left lung. Of unknown origin. Words I would come to hear far too often. Words that I would learn to question each time they were uttered. Words I would learn to hate.

The first diagnosis was BAC, or bronchioloalveolar carcinoma (a type of non-small cell lung cancer), joined by an unusual companion, mesothelioma. Both Stage IV, both incurable. It wasn't easy believing I had cancer, and incurable cancer at that. I didn't have any symptoms and I felt fine. *Surely they were wrong.* A diagnosis of pancreatic cancer came three years later and was equally as devastating in its prognosis.

How do you navigate through a triple cancer diagnosis and the resulting treatments all at the same time? How do you work with multiple doctors, different institutions, and a plethora of decisions that lead to seemingly endless possible outcomes? How do you keep your sanity in check?

How do you live a "normal" life? How do you deal with friends and loved ones? How do you know what to do next?

A CHANCE TO CHOOSE MY PATH

The short answer is: you don't. No one *tells* you, and no one hands you a manual with each contingency plan laid out in order. *If this happens, then you do this* . . . . Suggestions are made; *lots* of suggestions are made. But the hard reality is that the difficult decisions are left largely up to the patient, with little or no consistent basis on which to make those decisions. Each decision is a potential minefield, and every decision may close off options—options you might want to have in the future. In our current medical system when one has a fatal diagnosis, how fully informed is the patient, who must make the "right" decision? Well, that, too, is left up to the patient.

In this first-person account, I share my experiences regarding what I did, how I found information, how I tried to assess the potential usefulness of this information, and how I responded to unexpected detours along the way.

Read the choices I made, the questions I asked, the answers I sought, and the resources I used. Read with an eye for gaining tools for advocacy during treatment for yourself or a loved one. If you are in the medical profession, read to understand how the road looks from the other side of a deadly prognosis.

Based on my experiences, I highlight below some very specific ideas to keep in mind. Keep them handy, as they will help to give you some control over your medical treatment plan.

- Pay attention to your instincts. When the red flag waves in your mind, stop and ask yourself why. Then tell someone else.
- Have someone with you at doctors' appointments and through treatment. Your friends and loved ones are your best allies in treatment. They can listen with a more objective ear, and often they hear something you don't. Ask them to write down any ideas for later reference. Tomorrow might bring more clarity when you read it again.
- If you don't understand, *ask*. You are entitled to undivided attention and detailed explanations. It is up to you to make sure you get them.
- Even if you think you understand, ask again.
- Don't be put off by the jargon in medical reports. You don't have to understand all the medical terms to read reports about various tests. You can always look up definitions if you need to do so, but all you really need to know is what each medical scan or test is looking for and what it found.
- Join support groups in person, by email, by phone, or whatever works for you. Use them. Seek fellow-

ship of those who *understand* exactly what you are experiencing and who might have helpful suggestions because they may have similar experiences.

- When you feel as though you can't continue for one more minute, pray, cry, walk, hug someone, or stomp your feet. And then keep going. Your life depends on it.

Always remember: You are your own best advocate.

Read about my path as I traveled it, and take away what is helpful to you.

As of today, in mid-2013, both the pancreatic cancer and mesothelioma have returned. I started chemo yet again in what is very likely one last dance with fate.

The odds are against me, but they have been against me before, so I slog on. Whatever the outcome, I am grateful that I have always had a chance to choose my path through the medical minefield that typifies current cancer treatment.

INTRODUCTION:
PORTRAIT OF A LADY

I reveled in the extraordinary gift from my mother—a quarter at Northwestern University away from the College of Engineering, where I was enrolled. Neither she nor I were sure engineering had been a good choice for me, and now in 1960 I had spent three long years chafing under the demands of an engineering education with possible electives few and far between.

In the last two years of Northwestern's five-year engineering program, students were supposed to work somewhere in industry. Co-oping, it was called. Unfortunately, there didn't seem to be a great demand for "girl engineers" in the co-op ranks, and I wound up in a university research lab instead. The research was interesting, I enjoyed it and maybe even contributed a little something, but it wasn't like getting away, being off campus, doing something different.

So, the third time my co-op turn came around, I asked whether I could take some "interesting" courses instead. Probably annoyed with my choice of words, and maybe even with me, my engineering advisor said

I could do whatever I wanted to do but I had to keep paying tuition. That's when my mother stepped up to the plate.

With the entire university available to me, I opted for five upper-level classes: one in Shakespeare in the renowned Speech Department; a religion class; a writing seminar with Bergen Evans; a class in literature; and a three-times-a-week engaging slide show called Roman Archaeology. They were all classes for which I had none of the prerequisites. But, having only one semester away from "tech," there wasn't time to take any prerequisites, and it wasn't necessary, given Northwestern's recent switch to computerized registration.

Computerized registration in the early '60s meant you picked up pre-punched computer cards for the classes you wanted. Granted, there was a person who handed you the card and that person usually asked something like, "Have you had the prerequisites for this class?" A smile and a nod got me the card all five times, and in exchange, I turned in one of my registration cards with my name and particulars on it. These registration cards were color-coded. Different schools had different colors. The Technological Institute was orange.

None of the question-askers indicated that my orange cards were in any way unusual. They were more focused on the first part of the interaction: the question about prerequisites.

Unfortunately, it turns out that the question was a bit different for Professor Evans's seminar. Apparently, the lady asked, "Do you have permission to take this seminar?" I didn't notice this nuance, so I smiled and nodded, and got my card.

Of course, I didn't have permission. When I arrived at the once-a-week seminar, there was one more person than the venerable Bergen Evans had invited. And he knew who it was right away. In fact, he had my registration card in his hand. I'll never forget his waving the orange computer card in my direction and bellowing: "Miss Temple, I have never seen an orange card before. Just exactly what school are you enrolled in?"

He bellowed further when I confessed to being a stray engineer, and he told me to see him after class. It was a writing seminar, and I enjoyed the first class. I also thought that this first two hours was all I was going to get. But after class, Professor Evans told me I could stay for three weeks and, after that, if he didn't think I belonged, I had to agree to drop the class. I agreed.

It worked out quite well. I got to stay in the class, and when I graduated in 1961 with a B.S. in Engineering Physics, Bergen Evans managed to send me off to graduate school at Columbia University. His recommendation to Columbia's Graduate School of Journalism began: "Ignore the engineering degree, this young woman is a writer."

That semester was the best I had at Northwestern. All my classes were interesting. I could lie in bed, read, and think. I didn't have to be surrounded by a bunch of reference books, steam tables, slide rules, and their ilk. The thing I liked best, I think, was that there were no wrong answers. (No right ones either.) My interpretation of Lady Macbeth's "out damned spot" speech was a trial for me and doubtless the rest of the class, but by the end of the term I had learned enough about "interpretation" to merit a B. In fact, I think I got Bs in four of the five classes and an A in Roman Archaeology. Not bad for an engineer with no prerequisites!

The reading load was high but fascinating. The only book I put aside that semester was James's *Portrait of a Lady*. I found myself so moved by his writing that I couldn't read more than a few pages at a time. After those few pages, I spent many more minutes marveling at the words he chose and the mood he painted—in short, the sheer glory of his writing.

Finally, I decided that I didn't have time to actually read *Portrait of a Lady*. Instead, I forced myself to skim the book, barely getting what I needed for class and not dwelling on the actual words. I packed the book away with the conscious thought, "I want to really read this book someday, someday when I have time, someday before I die."

The book has moved with me many times over the last 53 years, always waiting on the bookshelf. Yesterday, I decided now was surely the time to finally revel in a careful reading of *Portrait of a Lady*. I took the old, red book down from the shelf, dusted it off, and started to read. James is certainly much better reading than the cancer poster papers, abstracts, and journals I've been slogging through for the last six years.

CHAPTER ONE

A STEEP LEARNING CURVE

X rays before a scheduled routine knee surgery in June 2006 revealed "anomalies of unknown origin" in my left lung. The nodules were diagnosed as "in keeping with probably ongoing inflammatory process," and I was treated for "probable pneumonia." But two rounds of antibiotics later, the spots were still there. A CT (computed tomography) scan (often called a "cat" scan) revealed the possibility of a recurrence of the breast cancer I had beaten twenty-six years ago, so it was time to start finding answers.

A SECOND OPINION

I had a preliminary follow-up CT scan in August, this time at National Jewish Health (NJH) in Denver. I met for the first time with pulmonologist Dr. David Buether, a man who would become my rock and my champion for years to come. He carefully reviewed the new scan and compared it to the existing films from Boulder Community Hospital (BCH) from two months before. The BCH scan report had the wrong date, so it appeared that Dr. Buether was comparing scans that were six *months* apart when they actually were barely six *weeks* apart. *Does this matter?* This was a question I would come to ask more and more over the months and years ahead: *Something is different—does this matter?*

Reading my reports was scary. In the latest one, the radiologist concluded that most of the nodules were "probably" larger than in the previous scan. Scariest of all, there was now a pleural "effusion" where there was only a pleural "irregularity" before. That is, now there was excess fluid in the pleural sac around my left lung.

The latest report ended with a seven-item *Impression*. Number one addressed the lung nodules specifically:

> *Multiple lung nodules, most of them appear to be slightly larger, compared to previous exam and the largest nodule is well defined and measured as 22.8 mm and located in the left lower lobe anterior segment.*

As I was soon to discover is often the case, the report concluded with a caveat that allowed me to overlook the entire summary, should I choose to do so.

It should be noted that measurements made on the comparison hard copy films are less accurate and therefore any perceived change in size of nodules may be less accurate.

This report sounded much worse than what I'd been told on the telephone when Dr. Buether said, "It's not reassuring in that the nodules have not gotten smaller. But it is reassuring that they have not gotten larger. So we're still in this limbo-land." He seemed greatly relieved that in September I was going for a check-up to MD Anderson Cancer Center (MDACC) in Houston, where I had been successfully treated for breast cancer in 1980. My suspicion was that he thought whatever was in my lungs was cancer and hoped it was not.

When reading scan reports, don't worry about understanding all the jargon. Any radiologist's report first presents a *Summary* of what was observed, followed by a section called *Impression*, which is where the radiologist discusses the conclusion about what the problem could be. Last is the *Findings*, in which the radiologist cites hard data, such as measurements and any noted changes. Read it all. If you have a previous scan, read it and carefully compare the scans. Is something mentioned in one but not the other? Does it matter? Make notes and ask your doctor.

TRYING TO LIVE NORMALLY

I was scared. I tried to work on my second mystery novel, *See How They Shine*, forcing myself to write maybe 500 words a day. They were not very interesting words because I wasn't sure of the plot yet. But my mind was elsewhere: *Do I have cancer? Is there some other explanation for all of this?*

I kept searching for answers on the Internet, but why was I doing that? What I could find wasn't encouraging, so it seemed dumb to continue searching. I couldn't find much good about the pleural effusion that had shown up on my latest scan. Mostly there were just cancer references.

The background humming in my brain about a possible diagnosis of cancer continued unabated. So much so that I called Rotary House in Houston, the full-service hotel available to MD Anderson patients and their families, and extended our reservation for an extra week after my September check-up and scan, should it become necessary. I had already arranged in-home care for B.J., our sweet, recently rescued, aging Labrador retriever. I also spent a lot of time getting "what if" commitments from friends so that B.J. could still stay home if we were in Houston for longer than we had planned.

A *THIRD* OPINION

Three weeks later, in September 2006, I was at MD Anderson in Houston for another round of scans, including a PET (positron emission tomography) scan. PET scans use a radioactive sugar solution to highlight areas of increased energy demand in the body. Areas using lots of sugar light up. Thus, the heart glows brightly on a PET scan. And so do tumors. Radiologists classify the degree of "glowing brightly" in units called SUVs (standard uptake values), which, as far as I could tell, were totally arbitrary and dimensionless numbers that allowed the radiologists to relate glow now to glow in the past in some perhaps meaningful numeric way. The radiologist's report stated: *"There is no evidence of FDG-avid disease."* (FDG is fluorodeoxyglucose, the radiopharmaceutical sugar.) The report further offered this *Impression*:

> *Multiple poorly marginated opacities in the lungs as well as the right upper lobe nodular opacity showing very low FDG uptake. This may be a pattern more in keeping with a chronic inflammatory process than metastatic disease. Given the lack of progression in the interval, a benign etiology such as chronic inflammation is favored. However, low-grade malignancy such as BAC could not be completely excluded. Tissue diagnosis may be*

helpful. Follow-up evaluation with CT
scanning may be necessary to assess the sta-
bility of these lesions.

The *Findings* section still included:

The largest nodule . . . in the left lower lobe
measuring 2.3 cm and stable in size compared
to prior exam . . . continues to demonstrate
low level FDG uptake with maximal SUV of
3.1.

A little worried, I read through to the end of the report:

Multiple, poorly marginated, noncalcified
nodules, the one in the right upper lobe meas-
uring approx. 1 cm; and one in left lower lobe
with SUV 1.9. Additionally there is another in
left lower lobe with SUV of 4. The most prom-
inent poorly marginated opacities (seen in
both lungs) have a maximum SUV of 1.2 in
keeping with probably ongoing inflammatory
process.

   What did this really mean? Some research papers said
anything with an SUV lower than 2.5 should be safe—not
cancer, but something else, such as inflammation. Others
argued that there is really no safe SUV level. And still
others mentioned the unsettling fact that the particular
kind of lung cancer known as BAC (bronchioloalveolar

carcinoma, the nonsmokers' lung cancer) is dismayingly "dark." In other words, it can have reassuringly low SUVs.

In the *Findings*, the radiologist mentioned a nodule in the lower lobe of my left lung with an SUV of 4, yet the *Impression* section made no specific mention of my left lower lobe, instead citing "no evidence of . . . disease." Perhaps this nodule glowing brightly at 4 SUV in my left lower lobe was covered by "multiple poorly marginated opacities." Worth a question at the very least.

FOLLOW-UP TESTING

Follow-up tests continued for months while pulmonologists from the country's number one cancer institution (MD Anderson) and leading lung disease institution (National Jewish) reassured me via email that there was nothing serious to worry about. I was told that the 2-cm lung nodule now appeared "slightly smaller," but the poorly defined, patchy GGO (ground-glass opacity) of the left lower lobe remained "unchanged and measures 26 mm."

So why was I still worried? I went on with my life . . . sort of. Instead of being my former workaholic self, I wasted time. I played a lot of solitaire on the computer. I dawdled on the manuscripts I was writing. It was as though I were daring fate to cut my time short. But, even as I wasted time, occasional unwelcome thoughts surfaced.

I would read an obituary and think, *mine will be there soon . . . I'd better write it.* I would do something and wonder whether it would be for the last time, or I would order tickets and contemplate whether I'd be here to use them.

Then there was my water jug from Lourdes—the one they sell in France with the picture of Mary on it. It was still there, full of the water I poured into it in 1981. It had protected me all these years. Was it failing me now? I would think, *well, everyone has to die sometime.* I kept having this thought and kept pushing it away as I half-heartedly continued to not do things I "should" have been doing, such as writing.

I discovered that even though I had been eating junk food for weeks, I had lost weight. Thoughts pervaded my waking hours. *Has it started already? Unexplained weight loss?*

Then, suddenly, I got two nibbles on my first mystery novel, *See How They Scurry.* One was more than a nibble—it was a request for a rewrite, and a fairly easy rewrite. With a new deadline in front of me, I tore into the rewrite, all the while keeping my every-three-months appointment with the pulmonologists and scanners at both MD Anderson and National Jewish. But I also was waking up every morning with tummy torsion, a huge knot lodged in my stomach, no doubt produced by worry and apprehension.

STILL SEARCHING FOR THE ANSWER

At the end of March 2007, I had yet another series of scans at MD Anderson as well as an appointment to meet there with the breast cancer doctor who had been following my case for the last ten years, Dr. Karin Hahn. I not only didn't see her, I didn't even know I wasn't going to see her until I arrived in her clinic. Since she had been my primary physician at MD Anderson for a decade, this was, to say the least, a shock. I'd come all the way to Houston only to meet instead with the nurse practitioner, who gave me the most recent scan report. The report included a startling new finding:

> *A new area of GGO in the periphery of the right lower lobe shows low-grade FDG activity, SUV 3.8.*

This didn't seem to be so "low grade" to me, and furthermore, it was new. But the rest of the *Impression* seemed unalarming enough:

> *Multiple areas of GGO as well as tiny nodules in both lungs are stable; more solid looking 2.3 cm left lower lobe nodule . . . unchanged since prior study of Sept. 20, 2006, suggest benign etiology.*

A LESSON IN MANAGING MY OWN CARE

For the next few days after I returned to Boulder, I remained quietly concerned about this new area in a previously uninvolved lung. Needing reassurance, I contacted Dr. Scott E. Evans, my pulmonologist at MD Anderson, via email.

> *Hello Dr. Evans:*
>
> *I am writing to remind you to check on the radiology report of my PET/CT scan done on March 29. You looked at the scans but said to check back to see what a second set of eyes might have to add.*
>
> *After meeting with you, I saw the nurse practitioner in Dr. Hahn's clinic. She had a verbal report on the PET/CT scan that included a comment about a "new area" that lit up. She said this was "probably inflammation" and asked me about cough, fever, etc. (No cough, no fever . . .)*
>
> *So, I'm wondering if, indeed, this most recent PET/CT scan is unremarkable. Thank you for the time to respond.*
>
> *Joann*

Dr. Evans responded almost right away.

Joann,

I agree that all of the areas of FDG-uptake look like inflammation, which is why we're still just watching you. While I'd like to see no new areas of interest, I don't think this mandates additional PET follow-up. I am comfortable having you follow-up by CT in Denver based on these studies in comparison to your earlier images.

Dr. Evans

I forwarded this email exchange to Dr. Buether at National Jewish, offering to send him the scan if he had not yet received it from Dr. Evans. I told him that I hadn't seen Dr. Hahn when I was in Houston, so I didn't have her opinion on any of this.

I ended the email with my summary of the results as I understood them thus far: nothing in the existing nodules had changed, a new spot was probably inflammation, I should return for a follow-up scan at National Jewish in July and I should repeat my PET/CT scan at MD Anderson in a year.

Dr. Buether must have been sitting at his computer, as he responded quickly to my email.

Joann,

Thanks for your update. News sounds good. I don't know that you need frequent (or even any!) additional PET scans at this point. I would follow these nodules by CT scan every 3-6 months (you may consider 6 instead of 3 months because nodules have been stable for some time, and there is a risk to excessive radiation exposure from frequent CT scans). If MDACC feels it would help, I would consider a repeat PET in 1 year, but I don't know that you need a PET in 6 months, particularly given the expense and inconvenience you go through.

Again, if these were really small nodules there would be no question that their lack of growth implies they are benign. Their larger size makes all of us a bit more nervous, which has prompted all of the frequent scans. My experience with recurrent or metastatic cancer is that it doesn't grow slowly, although primary lung cancer does grow very slowly sometimes. We are trying to balance the risks of waiting too long (missing cancer) against the risks, inconvenience, worry, and expense of looking too frequently. If it was just one nodule, I would usually recommend surgical resection at this point so that we would be done with all of this. But that wouldn't help us here because of the other nodules.

Dave

CLARIFICATION, PLEASE

After hearing from both Dr. Evans and Dr. Buether, I asked Dr. Evans: "Do you think a CT here at National Jewish is sufficient for the next year?"

> *Joann,*
>
> *As I recall our discussion, I suggested six months as an appropriate follow-up date. You stated that you had planned a visit to National Jewish in July, and I replied that there was no convincing argument to be made for July vs. September. With the specter of a new FDG-avid area (admittedly a non-too-threatening specter), I might err toward keeping your scheduled July appointment—but I have no data to prove the wisdom of that recommendation.*
>
> *Dr. Evans*

Feeling as though I had been "blown off" by MD Anderson during my last visit when I failed in my attempt to see my breast cancer doctor despite having an appointment, I decided to keep Dr. Buether in the loop when I received an appointment schedule from MD Anderson with all sorts of tests and plans for my next visit proposed for October 2007.

Hi:

MDACC sent me an appointment schedule in-cluding a PET/CT (and a bunch of other tests but no MD appointments) for late October. I queried Dr. Evans and he replied that he didn't think I needed another PET/CT scan unless they were doing it for breast cancer surveillance.

I certainly don't want to go to Houston for a bunch of tests (blood work, mammogram, etc.), not see a physician there again, and then have to request the test results when I get home. (Am I being too snarky?)

So, unless this July CT shows some significant change, I hope to just cancel this October se-quence in Texas and stay home from now on. But, we should discuss that plan when I see you, I guess.

Thanks,

Joann

His answer:

Hi Joann,

I agree with your plan. The MDACC stuff sounds excessive to me too. You're not being snarky; just don't upset anyone over there too

*much because we never know if we might
need them in the future. But I'd save your
money and time for now, particularly if the
July CT looks OK. We'll talk more when I see
you, of course.*

Dave

UNLESS THERE IS SIGNIFICANT CHANGE . . .

It turned out that my words, "unless this July CT shows
some significant change," had been prophetic. There *was*
significant change. The doctors stopped calling the spot in
my left lung an "anomaly" and began calling it a "lesion."
Growth was confirmed by National Jewish. It was time for
a biopsy.

I discussed with both Dr. Buether and Dr. Evans the
need to undergo VATS (Video-Assisted Thoracoscopic
Surgery). Each doctor sought to reassure me why this invasive biopsy, which they had eschewed for so long, was
now necessary. The surgery would require three small incisions, one for the thoracoscope so the surgeon could see
inside the chest cavity and two more for surgical instruments. The surgery would require both anesthesia and
hospitalization.

Early in the morning of July 3, 2007, I received an email from Dr. Buether that laid out the situation from his perspective.

Joann,

There has been some variation, particularly of the ground-glass nodule, and that is partly due to the fact that ground-glass nodules aren't 100% solid, so they tend to vary more on imaging.

I spent some time yesterday afternoon with Dr. Newell, one of our thoracic radiologists. We really felt that the overall trend of your last few scans was one of slow growth. Yes, there have been some ups and downs in size, but overall, many of the nodules are clearly bigger—not dramatically, but now it is pretty clear they are growing.

I emailed Scott Evans at MDACC and he already replied to me (he's a quick one!). I told him I am concerned that we have no diagnosis for these growing nodules, so even though the PET scan is not overwhelmingly positive, I would recommend a biopsy. He agreed that bronchoscopy would be unlikely to yield a result. In talking with our radiologists, those two bigger nodules in the left lower lobe are challenging to get to with a CT-guided needle biopsy because the solid one is right next to the diaphragm (which means it moves a lot when you breathe), and because the ground-glass nodule is not dense, it is sometimes difficult to know whether or not you are in the ground-glass nodule.

In addition to that, while this could be infection or vasculitis, those two things usually cause you to feel sick/have a lot of symptoms. If it is slow-growing cancer, we might anticipate that the PET scan would be only weakly positive, and topping our list of potential diagnoses would be lymphoma, bronchioloalveolar cell carcinoma, and metastatic disease (breast or other). Those first two particularly are difficult to make a definitive diagnosis with the small amount of tissue we get with needle biopsies or bronchoscopy.

Based on all this, if it were me or a loved one going through this, I would have a surgical biopsy of these two nodules in the L[eft] lower lobe. We have some of the best thoracic surgeons in the world. They would likely recommend a limited procedure called VATS— Video Assisted Thoracoscopic Surgery. It would involve several small incisions, general anesthesia, and a 3-5 day hospital stay, with some discomfort related to the procedure, but would give us a much better idea of what these nodules are. I am fairly concerned about lymphoma—we haven't talked about that, but if that is what this is, it is quite treatable so I wouldn't want to wait another 6–12 months to find out.

Let me know your thoughts on all of this, when you are ready. If you want to come in and talk, we could do that too. The surgeons actually talk to you quite a bit about this procedure, too, if you want to proceed, which is unusual sometimes for surgeons. I don't want to push you into anything you don't want to do, but this is my recommendation as if I were in your shoes.

Dave

A couple of hours later, in answer to my inquiry about timing, and who the "we" was who had "some of the best thoracic surgeons," Dr. Buether responded to my email:

A lot to take in, but there is something to be said for not screwing around with a bunch of procedures that are unlikely to help you, and most people that go through VATS lung biopsy do very well. I am talking about [two thoracic surgeons at University of Colorado

*Health Sciences Center]. We work very close-
ly with them. All they do is lung surgery, 24/7.
Either one is excellent.*

*They usually can get you in very quickly. I
will have Joann (my nurse, your namesake)
work on getting you into their clinic. You typ-
ically would see them in clinic Monday, and if
all your questions are answered and they
don't need any more testing, they can often do
the procedure that same week. I imagine you
could get in and have your surgery by the end
of July, which is more than fast enough. Remember, these nodules are slow growing so if
it gets into early August, it isn't the end of the
world. But I imagine you want to take care of
this sooner rather than later. I'll get going on
this today.*

Dave

Five days later, I reported to Dr. Buether on my progress in scheduling an appointment with the surgeon at
University Hospital (UH—what everyone calls UCHSC). I
also asked a bunch of questions:

*I have an appointment with the thoracic sur-
geon at 3:30 Monday. I'll let you know how
that goes.*

*In gathering up all the reports and so forth
that I have, I tried to correlate the CT and*

PET/CT findings. This exercise has left me thoroughly befuddled. Even noting your caution about lack of repeatability, I still did this. What can I say? I'm an engineer at heart, I guess. I hope you can answer the following questions off the top of your head and not have to take time to look at the scans again. I do think it's a matter of terminology. So, here goes:

There are three GGOs in my left lung mentioned in every report but sited at four different locations—lower lateral, lower posterior, lower superior, and inferior lingula. [Lingula refers to a projection of the upper lobe of the left lung.]

Q#1. Are lower lateral and lower posterior the same place?

Q#2. If not, which are the same place in the above list of four locations? (Or are there four areas of GGO and only three are mentioned each time?)

Q#3. I really cannot correlate the last two CT scans done at NJH. The original report gives different numbers than those cited in the subsequent report and attributed to the earlier report. Is this because Dr. Newell went back and re-measured the earlier scan? The reason I would like to know the above is because, if I have figured out which measurement goes to which GGO, it appears to me that the largest GGO has the lowest SUV uptake of 1.7. If that's true, I am assuming that is NOT the GGO we propose to biopsy and I want to talk to the surgeon about the likelihood of successfully finding the smaller one (SUV 4.0 somewhere).

Q#4. Also, the solid nodule seems to be stable, allowing for differences in orientation. Do you know if it is proposed to biopsy that as well?

Q#5. Lastly, are we ignoring the changes in my right lung? I'm assuming biopsy on both lungs wouldn't happen at the same time.

Q#6. In the literature, I've seen various statements that suggest nodule size greater than 3 cm is a point for concern/action and that SUV lower than 2.5 is 100% indication of a benign process. Are these two statements correct?

I hope you have time to deal with these probably misguided questions before I see the surgeon Monday afternoon. (I'm saving up a bunch more questions for him and I expect I'd like to come back and talk to you again, bringing Roger this time.)

Thank you!

Joann

Dr. Buether gave a hurried response.

Joann,

I have to run, but basically if a nodule is getting larger, we aren't as concerned about what the PET says—there is no 100% indication that something is benign, and particularly when it is slow growing.

I think I would rather leave up to the surgeon which nodules he wants to biopsy. That is more dependent upon what is technically best for you and him, and may even be a decision made in the operating room. Let's see what this shows first before worrying about the right side. If left-sided biopsies don't give us a diagnosis, we may follow this or go after the new right nodule if it doesn't go away.

It is difficult to impossible to look at all of these reports and make sense of this, but when you look at the images serially, it is clear many of the nodules are slowly growing, and that is why we are here.

Dave

At this point, I was still concerned about the wisdom of an invasive biopsy and asked Dr. Evans for his opinion.

Hello Dr. Evans:

I know you have talked with Dr. Buether at NJH about my most recent (and previous) CT scans there. Dr. Buether is recommending a biopsy but acknowledges that another six months of watchful waiting is an option.

After talking with the thoracic surgeon at the University of Colorado Hospital today, I am, frankly, concerned that a biopsy is going to permanently impair me while possibly still not providing a definitive diagnosis.

This leads me to try to weigh the risk of biopsy vs. the risk of more watchful waiting. Are you willing to have an opinion on that question? And, if you think the risk substantial, do you think I should have the biopsy done at MDACC?

Thank you for thinking about these two questions. (I am copying Dr. Buether on the content of this email).

Joann

Dr. Evans promptly replied with a thoughtful email.

Dear Mrs. Dennett:

You seem to have correctly surmised that there is no absolute correct answer to your question. However, we have been engaged in a watchful waiting for some time, and are now faced with non-reassuring findings (rather than stability or resolution of the findings).

So, it seems that both Dr. Buether and I feel compelled to proceed with biopsy. We don't want to miss a malignancy—lymphoma and bronchioloalveolar lung cancer are the two that jump to mind with your scans—after following for this long.

As for the location, I indicated to Dr. Buether that I would support your decision for either center. MDACC and NJH offer similarly excellent services (something I can't say for many patients' local hospitals), and I don't think I can make a terribly strong recommendation either way. If the biopsy were positive for cancer, then Dr. Buether has already indicated he'd expect you'll want to come back here. If you'd prefer to be here so that (1) our extremely adept cancer pathologists are able to see the samples right away, or (2) you'd like to see an oncologist sooner after a potential cancer diagnosis, then I'm happy to arrange the biopsy for you. However, there's a lot to be said for convenience to you and your family, and the general comfort of being close to home. Again, I'll support either choice without hesitation.

I think you might be overestimating the potential impairment associated with the procedure. I'd rather use a less invasive approach, but they should still be able to use video assisted surgery to minimize wounds, hospital stay, discomfort, etc. I don't want to minimize your (appropriate) concerns, but I anticipate few long-term complications. If I did, I'd wait till these lesions grew larger to biopsy them some other way.

In summary: (1) we can watch a bit longer, but both of your pulmonologists think this is a less-than-ideal option, (2) the choice of center for the biopsy is truly yours, with each having unique benefits but no real downside, (3) while not entirely pleasant, the surgical biopsy is not expected to result in long-term problems. Hope this helps. Feel free to contact me with further questions.

Scott E. Evans, M.D.

I then sent him one "last" question regarding whether, if I had the biopsy in Denver and if it were cancer, he could arrange for me to get into the MD Anderson system quickly. He replied, again right away: "Yes, I am happy to arrange evaluation on this end."

I copied Dr. Buether on the emails with Dr. Evans and asked yet further questions, adding that I just was trying not to be in a position in a month or so where I wished I'd asked more questions.

> *Hi:*
>
> *Here's what Dr. Evans had to say. The only thing that was a new thought to me was that, if the anomalies get bigger, they are easier to sample less invasively. Is that true with the location of my nodules?*
>
> *And, if it is true, there is obviously some risk in waiting for them to grow . . . more so with BAC than with lymphoma, I think. Is BAC even treatable beyond resection?*
>
> *My MAJOR concern with the biopsy is that I really cannot imagine getting through it without getting pneumonia . . . given my apparent proclivity for doing so.*
>
> *Joann*

Dr. Buether's reply was almost immediate:

Non-resectable BAC is treatable, but not curable. Nodules would have to grow quite a bit for less invasive techniques to be preferable to VATS, and waiting is less than ideal. And VATS allows us to sample more than one. For most patients, VATS biopsy isn't that traumatic and rarely results in long-term problems. The person doing your surgery is extremely good at this procedure (one of the best in the country, really), and that is worth a lot in terms of how you do, and how good the information is that we get. Your pneumonia risk is real, but not much more than someone without lung disease, and presumably we'd be keeping a close eye on you and treating early and aggressively, preventing that from being anything more than a minor setback.

Dave

SCHEDULING THE VATS BIOPSY

Convinced that I should go ahead with the VATS biopsy at UH, I inquired of Dr. Buether about the logistics of scheduling it.

Seriously, I realize I have to do this and am now trying to sort out what I have to get done, what I can offload onto someone else and/or delay substantially and who I owe what beforehand. . . . I do think I need to wait until second summer term is over, given that I promised an unwell colleague that I would be available should she need help. So, I'm thinking August 2 or 6.

The surgeon operates on Tuesdays and Fridays. I suppose there is something to be said in favor of Friday surgery and weekend hospitalization as opposed to Tuesday surgery and maybe being home on the weekend. (I'm still fixated on the pneumonia issue . . . probably will be until this is over.)

Joann

Dr. Buether's reply:

Either day is fine. I like Tuesday because there are more people around if you have problems the 1-2 days after, and you are home on the weekend. But the hospital is 24/7, and it doesn't really matter.

Dave

I decided that August 7, 2007, would be the best date for me, and I started to make the necessary arrangements. The first arrangement turned out to be to change the date to one that the surgeon could make, which was Friday, August 10.

In preparation for the surgical biopsy, I questioned Dr. Buether about the results of the cumulative scans, specifically about why so suddenly things were "clearly larger" when before they had been mostly stable or smaller.

> *Hi:*
>
> *One last question. On re-reading the CT reports, I realized that, until this time, the comments were mostly that things were stable or smaller. Now, in a six-month interval, they are "clearly larger." How dependent, if at all, is that judgment on my body position during the scan? I ask because, on the day of the last CT scan, I was experiencing a lot of shoulder pain when I raised my right arm. Accordingly, I was unable to extend that arm above my head as usual and wound up having to rest my hand on my head with my elbow pointed forward during the scan. Comparing the two arm positions today at home, it is clear that the expansion of my chest is certainly different on the right and maybe so on the left.*
>
> *If there is any possibility this would have produced anomalous results, should we repeat the CT scan?*
>
> *Joann*

You may have to ask the radiologist to look farther back in time than the last scan. Do it. It could be important.

Slight differences scan-to-scan can be significant in the long run, but growth or changes are easier to see on scans farther apart in time. Often the scan reports suspicious spots in two dimensions. Remember, a small change in width (diameter) could be a large change in volume.

There was a lot of truth in his response to my email—truth that was never before explicitly stated to me but is important to understand.

Joann,

Because of this issue of variation in position, technique, or the amount of inflammation that surrounds a nodule, when nodules are slightly bigger the scan can often be read out as "no change," so as not to cause undue alarm when the size is truly the same. The next time they might be slightly smaller. In the past your scans that have shown "no change" have really shown slight growth in the nodules, and that is really only evident in retrospect, looking serially at all of your scans. If you only compare to the most recent scan every time, you can write off slight increase as no significant change every time (particularly if the PET is reassuringly negative), and if you don't periodically look back at the trend over multiple scans you can miss slow growth.

Also, a small change in nodule diameter translates into a large change in nodule volume, particularly for these bigger 2-cm nodules.

Dave

WAITING FOR THE VATS BIOPSY

I grew more concerned about the biopsy as the surgery date drew near, and I continued to question Dr. Buether by email.

Dr. Buether,

In our meeting with the surgeon, he said that everything would be re-explained. On that premise, I did not press him on several questions that he didn't really answer. Now, in reviewing my pre-op schedule, I don't see any place on it where I will confer further with him at any substantive length. So, I'd like to ask you a few more questions please.

First, when are the biopsy results available? Specifically, do they affect what happens in surgery? Frozen section and then try to remove malignancy, if there is one? (I ask this obviously from my experience with a breast biopsy in 1980.) I did ask the surgeon this and his answer focused on what labs got what,

*what they did with it, and how very competent
they are. He did not address what might happen in surgery and, as noted above, I chose
not to repeat my question.*

*Second, if this is a malignancy, I would like to
consult MDACC before any further treatment
in order to keep all my options open. I did
NOT discuss this with the surgeon specifically, but he mentioned that, if it were malignant,
"we would all" be caring for me. I'm not sure
how we got to that point in the discussion, but
I certainly hope you are in that "we" somewhere. Are you?*

*If not, I want someone to be aware of my
preference to at least consult Dr. Evans and
whatever oncologist he suggests at MDACC
before proceeding with any treatment here.
Who should that "someone" be? (I'm assuming that I may not be in any shape to ask such
questions or advocate for myself on such issues immediately.)*

Joann

Dr. Buether remained ever diligent and patient with his
responses to my questioning:

Joann,

*Many of these questions are better answered
by the surgeon and his team.*

Final pathology results take 2–3 days, sometimes more. In the case of an isolated nodule, the usual practice is to do frozen section in the OR and if it is cancer, do the definitive resection. Your situation is different. You have many nodules. Lymphoma requires a diagnosis and chemotherapy, not a larger resection, for example. And since there are several nodules, it isn't clear that the same process is responsible for all of them, nor would this approach of "if it's cancer, take it all out" necessarily make sense.

So I don't know the OR plan exactly, but I imagine it will be more about getting a diagnosis than cutting a lot out. Hopefully, this is all benign, but if it is metastatic cancer, we would recommend going to MDACC (we are aware of your preferences), and surgery may not be the next step. Most likely, this will all be a discussion that occurs after you have recovered from your surgery and we have pathology back. Hopefully, it is a discussion about how they aren't cancer.

Hang in there—I know this is a difficult time for you.

Dave

The day before the VATS, I expressed my concern to Dr. Buether about getting the results of the biopsy as soon as possible:

> *Dr. Buether,*
>
> *I met with the surgeon again today preparatory to the biopsy tomorrow afternoon. He is a very careful listener, which I appreciated.*
>
> *He told me that the biopsy results would be available "when I see him for follow up" some days after surgery. I asked if you would receive the results also. I believe he said that you would if they were relevant to you (not his exact words).*
>
> *In any event, I do want you to get the biopsy results and I do want to know what they are as soon as possible, particularly if they need to be communicated to Dr. Evans.*
>
> *So, I'm hoping you can help me with timely information. I will mention this to the surgeon again also.*
>
> *Thank you,*
>
> *Joann*

THE FIRST OF MANY BIOPSIES

Surgery day, August 10, 2007, began with a phone call from University Hospital in Aurora asking whether I could come in early, like right now. This was about nine in the morning, and as I wasn't scheduled until much later, I had finished my last cup of coffee only an hour earlier. I conveyed this information to the nurse and was told, "That's okay, it doesn't matter."

Really? It doesn't matter? Then why do they always ask you not to eat or drink for hours before surgery if it doesn't matter? Interesting.

In any event, since we live almost fifty miles from University Hospital, there wasn't any "right now" about it. We got there as soon as we could, which was closer to eleven than ten. I was whisked right in and prepped. The anesthesiologist came by, and I lamented the fact that it had taken me more than twenty-four hours to get warm again after my two previous surgeries. She told me that the operating room was *always* cold, but when she left, she said she would turn the heat up. She must have done so because it was the first surgery that I came out of feeling warm. In fact, all things about the surgery were better than usual. All things, that is, except the news given to me in the recovery room.

POSTSURGERY

After getting my attention as I was coming out of anesthesia, a physician who was present in the operating room said something to the effect of, "You remember we did this surgery because we had a suspicion of cancer? We still have that suspicion." I went back to sleep and the next thing I knew, my bed was being pushed off an elevator. It took some maneuvering, but finally we were off the elevator and en route to my room.

Roger and a family friend were in my room when I got there. Unfortunately, my few lucid moments in the recovery room seemed to have provided more information about the surgery than either of them had received. Roger hadn't heard the cell phone ring when the operating room called to say that the surgeon was ready to talk to him. Giving a waiting family a cell phone is a wonderful innovation, but they should also be sure the ringer is loud enough for old folks to hear it.

Knowing little about the results of the operation, we instead discussed the hospital, my room, and the view. University Hospital had been in its new home in Aurora less than two weeks. The room was spacious, comfortable, and full of light. There was even a full-size couch for overnight guests.

Roger was staying the first night, and we had other volunteers lined up to stay for subsequent nights, should they be needed. Alas, they were indeed needed. I called them my in-room advocates. The hospital apparently agreed to some degree with the concept of in-room advocates because they provided clean linen each night for my overnight visitors.

MY IN-ROOM ADVOCATES

The too-soft-to-hear cell phone was but one example of a great new idea poorly implemented. Meal service was another. Hardly a new idea, but to say it was poorly implemented would be an understatement. The first day, of course, I got the usual postsurgery diet of not much. Two days later, I was looking forward to real food, even though I was on restricted fluids and low salt due to latent heart issues.

I was therefore quite surprised to see my breakfast: a huge Belgian waffle, bacon, coffee, and juice. "I can't eat this. It's not what I ordered!" I blurted out, not thinking to be diplomatic. The answer I got, however, was stupefying. My meal-delivery person who had brought the tray in and taken the metal cover off of the hot food with such a flourish put her hands on her hips and said, "Did you fax your order to the kitchen?"

> Every hospital patient needs an in-room advocate these days—an extra set of ears, eyes, and legs. You are likely to need help in unpredictable ways.
>
> Many hospitals provide beds and bedding for your in-room advocate. If such accommodations are not obvious, ask for them.

Speechless, I could only stare at her. My overnight in-room advocate, a longtime friend from church, grabbed my tray and demanded, "Take me to the kitchen."

Off they went, and soon she was back with a tray full of food I could eat. She reported encountering another patient in full gown regalia pushing his IV (intravenous) pole toward the kitchen and muttering about the lack of coffee, let alone food. She also had a menu for the rest of Sunday and Monday. I filled it out, and off she went to find a fax machine.

Later that day, another good friend who shared my love of opera arrived to spend the night. She brought along a tape of one of Peter Sellars' Mozart operas, *Cosi Fan Tutte*. We stayed up way too late watching this hilarious production. I finally cut the evening off, knowing the X-ray people would be in at five in the morning to see if the air leak from the surgery was gone from my lung yet. So, we saved the last act for the next day and amused the CNA (certified nursing assistant) with our enjoyment of such a "weird" art form.

I saw the surgeon each day, and each day he checked the level of fluids still oozing out of my side. If air bubbles were still visible, it meant that the incision in my lung hadn't yet closed. I wound up staying an extra day in the hospital until the air leak had stopped to his satisfaction.

So five days after surgery, I was finally ready to go home, not yet knowing what had been discovered, but hoping it was a treatable lymphoma. The nurse went over my discharge papers with Roger and me and called "transportation" to get me to the car. Roger took my things and went off to find the car while I waited until a lady with a wheelchair showed up. She and I set off for the front door via the elevator but, just as the doors began to close, another patient in a wheelchair arrived. Since the elevator buttons were at eye level from my wheelchair, I hit the "open door" button and the second wheelchair was pushed aboard.

I thought nothing about this until we were exiting the elevator on the ground floor. The transport person for the second wheelchair said to the woman who was pushing me, "I heard what you said about me, bitch, and I'm waiting for you." She then did a quasi-wheelie with her patient and went off in the opposite direction from where we seemed to be heading.

"Good grief!" I said to the woman who I had begun to think of as "my lady."

"She's nuts, that girl. I don't know what she's talking about," was the answer as my wheelchair seemed to pick up speed toward the hospital entrance.

It took Roger a few more minutes to get the car through the traffic jam at the entrance and, when he did so, there were two other cars between us and him. I pointed out our van, and "my lady" pushed me off the sidewalk, weaving around between the parked cars to get to the side of our van.

Just as I put my hand on the van door, ready to get out of the wheelchair, the other attendant appeared right in front of me. The expression on her face was scary and her words were scarier as she spoke to "my lady."

"I told you, bitch, I'm right over there. Waiting for you."

I stood up, slid into the van, and slammed the door. "My lady" turned the wheelchair and took off the way we had come. The second woman was still standing there when we pulled away.

An hour or so later, we got home. I felt amazingly good but was anxious about the biopsy, the results of which I expected any day. Silly, silly me.

AWAITING THE RESULTS OF THE BIOPSY

I spent the first five days at home trying to get information about the biopsy results. My frustration was mounting, and I emailed Dr. Buether.

> *Dr. Buether,*
>
> *I don't really know anything yet except that the nodule was not in my lung but on my diaphragm. I've asked the surgeon to let me know about the pathology as soon as he knows. I will then attempt to forward that info to Dr. Evans in Houston.*

I guess I may also know the following. (1) In addition to the nodule in/on the diaphragm, there were two similar-appearing lesions on the chest wall. The surgeon sent one for frozen section and got back "suspicious for tumor." He then removed the large nodule. (I don't know about the other one.) (2) The surgeon thought the lung tissue looked maybe okay but that the lesions on the chest wall/diaphragm looked like metastases. (3) In the Recovery Room, the Fellow said something to the effect of "We did this surgery because of a suspicion of cancer. We still have that suspicion."

Also, there seems to have been some puzzlement over where my records are. Specifically, the diagnostic radiologist lamented not having access to previous CT scans or X rays. On 08/12, Roger gave all the X rays from University Family Medicine to the X-ray tech who came to my room to do the morning chest X ray. So, radiology should have all the X rays. I don't know whether they still want the CT scans but, if they do, can you possibly tell them how/where to find the CT scans online?

Thank you,

Joann

At the same time, I also sent an email to my primary care physician at University Family Medicine in Boulder.

I am writing this for four reasons.

First, I had the VATS biopsy a week ago and am waiting for the path results. I don't really know anything yet except that the nodule was not in my lung but on my diaphragm. I've asked the surgeon to let me know about the pathology as soon as he knows. (His first response to that request was that he would tell me when he sees me on August 27. After I objected about such a long delay, he indicated that he would call me when he had the results.) The results should be available today, I think. He is in surgery on Fridays so I don't know if I will hear from him before next week or not. (Meantime, I am trying not to go crazy . . . but it's not working very well.)

Second, the diagnostic radiologist at UH wanted the X rays from University Family Medicine. On 08/12, Roger gave all the X rays that I had from University Family Medicine to the X-ray tech who came to my hospital room to do the morning chest X ray. I hope this means the X rays are back in the system and not lost, but . . . .

Third, every time I saw paperwork at UH, it listed Lonnie Granston as my primary care physician. I tried, every time I saw this, to get this changed to you. They kept saying it didn't matter. I certainly want you to get information/results etc. Do I need to do anything to achieve that?

Fourth, I am supposed to get the path results to MDACC as soon as possible. They should include my MDACC patient number. I can do this, once I get the path results.

Thank you, Joann

For several more days, the surgeon continued to remain mum on the biopsy results. I sent an email to him on August 17, 2007, just to remind him that I existed, and asking about taking daily low-dose aspirin. I received no reply to that email, either.

The following email exchange with Dr. Buether a few days later underscores the frustration I was experiencing.

Dr. Buether,

On Friday, the surgeon indicated he might have results Saturday. It is Monday at 10 am, I have heard nothing from anyone, and I know that the surgeon sees patients in the office on Monday. (So he's probably not reading email.)

I am getting really anxious about this. It has been 6 weeks since the CT scan that showed things were growing. The nodules weren't in my lungs but diaphragm/chest wall. They're trying to differentiate the "type of tumor." It could take two or more weeks to get appointments with an oncologist, either here or at MDACC. It all sounds, to me, as though I need to be in a screaming hurry.

My past experience (which is considerable) with bad news pathology is that doctors are reluctant to just give patients the information without a face-to-face meeting. I don't see the surgeon for another week, by which time I will have taken all of my dog's remaining thunderstorm valium.

Can you possibly shake loose ANY information? Should we tell Dr. Evans at this point that the nodule wasn't in my lung? (Depending on what types of tumor they are trying to differentiate among, that could mean that he can't help me at MDACC and I have to wend my way through a different administrative labyrinth down there.)

In short, I am losing it in this information vacuum.

Joann

Dr. Buether couldn't make things speed along, but he could offer empathy.

Joann,

I am sorry you are going through this. The pathologists are doing some special stains to determine what type of tumor. As you suggest, that is very important in terms of the next step for you. It wouldn't hurt to let MDACC know what is going on, but I think it would be better to have all the information in hand when you contact them, and the surgeon should know something more definitive tomorrow, after which you can proceed.

I don't know if that was helpful. If this is metastatic cancer, sometimes that is very difficult to characterize in more detail by just looking at it under the microscope, and requires special stains, and even then can be difficult to pin down exactly. But oncologists are not unfamiliar with this situation, and can develop an appropriate treatment plan even when there is some uncertainty with the pathology results. But we will need the final pathology report first.

Dave

FINALLY, THE RESULTS

The surgeon finally called the next day, August 20, ten days after the VATS. I wasn't at home. He told Roger just that I have two cancers and I should call him back.

I thought, *Call a surgeon? Ha!* I finally prevailed on my primary care physician, who was in the UH system, to see if the biopsy report had been posted. She faxed it to me.

The biopsy had turned up not one, but two primary cancers: one in my lung, the other on my diaphragm and chest wall. The diagnosis was BAC and mesothelioma. Both Stage IV, both incurable.

My primary care physician called me, so distressed by the diagnosis that she broke into tears when she affirmed the answer to my question, "Meso's a matter of only months, isn't it?"

During those ten harrowing days from surgery to pathology results, many people called or emailed, some repeatedly, asking whether I had the results. Now I did have the results: two deadly cancers.

With the help of a friend who had taken on the role of my right-hand woman through all of this, I had compiled an email list asking everyone to hold off with their questions and promising to let them know when I knew. She kept that promise with the following email, sent on August 21, 2007:

Dear Family and Friends of Joann,

Joann got the pathology report today and it is devastating. She has two kinds of cancer: Mesothelioma and BAC (bronchioloalveolar carcinoma). This is highly unusual and there may be no treatment protocols for the mixture. Mesothelioma is the immediate threat. Its median survival is 12.5 months. She is in contact with a research doctor at MDACC who says he will get her into the system there ASAP.

This is a physician (Jon Kurie) whose work Joann has written about over the years. He is not her physician, but he is a full professor at UT/MDACC. He seems to care about Joann— he answered her first email in two minutes— and she believes he will help her get to the right people in a timely manner. Although she fears that there is probably nothing to be done, she is still hopeful that MDACC will have some good ideas and that those good ideas can be implemented at the new cancer center in Boulder. She really doesn't want to go back and forth to Texas repeatedly and, in fact, doesn't want to go back and forth to University Hospital in Aurora repeatedly.

*So, in short, Joann is in shock, trying to find a
good course of action, doing something, and,
unfortunately for those of us who would love
to talk to her, not wanting to talk about it! Also, her brother-in-law, Donald, and his
friend, Peg, arrive tomorrow for a week. They
know that Roger and Joann may be leaving
for Texas. The present plan is to drive.*

*If you've got any good ideas, please email Jo-
ann. In fact, any kind of email is okay, just
don't expect her to talk to you about this pathology until she has some idea what to say.*

Please, please don't call her.

Thank you.

CHOOSING THE NEXT STEP

Poking around online later that month, I met a fellow patient through the Boulder Public Library's Grillo Health
Information Center. His diagnosis was similar to mine: two
uniformly fatal cancers. We were roughly the same age
and both held PhDs; hence, our mutual, common struggle
to gather, filter, and assess information was underpinned
by confidence in the scientific method.

My online friend had completed six cycles of chemotherapy with good success. In the words of his oncologist,

"the disease was savaged." No evidence of the disease remained after chemo. His expectation, and that of his physicians, was that the cancers would return in nine to twelve months. So, he started looking for "Plan B." After returning from a consultation at Dana Farber at Harvard University, he wrote that his primary oncologist advocated Cyberknife, a noninvasive robotic radiosurgery system, not really a knife. The oncologist at Harvard, however, disagreed and suggested taking Tarceva, a relatively new chemotherapeutic pill that had the potential of achieving prolonged remission. The Harvard physician also argued that there were immediate synergistic drug choices available if Tarceva began to fail. My email friend summed up his dilemma well:

> The choice of cancer treatment, such as it is, is largely up to the patient. When one has a fatal diagnosis in our current medical system, final decisions on treatment are often left up to the patient. How informed can that decision be? That, too, is left up to the patient.
>
> This is the bottom-line problem for the cancer patient. You have to make your own decisions. And you have little or no basis on which to make those decisions. Yet every decision is a potential minefield. Every decision may close off other options— options you might want to have in the future.

Not only do cancer patients with a poor prognosis have to wrestle physically with their disease but also must make possible life and death choices among the views of differing oncologists.

Trying to be helpful in my friend's dilemma, I unearthed an abstract about post-chemo Cyberknife results on twelve patients who had Stage IIIB or Stage IV lung cancer. It reported relatively positive results, but, when I forwarded it to him, I added that I tend to whistle in the dark. He closed his reply email with the following:

> *Hey, if we are going to be mutually supportive, then if you decide to plunge off into the darkness to confront our common demons, shouldn't I at least follow behind holding a flashlight?*

"Holding a flashlight" seems to be all most physicians are willing to do for terminal patients. Deciding where to point the flashlight would be more helpful.

CHAPTER TWO

A WHOLE NEW CAST OF PLAYERS

Every day I awoke with the thought, *Soon, soon I am going to die. I don't want to die.* I for sure didn't want to die as ugly a death as mesothelioma seemed to promise. I still had thirty-nine of the forty Dilaudid pills prescribed for VATS pain. I reflected: *Is that enough? Will I know when to do it? Will I be able to?* Not the best time to explore theological issues, I decided.

Then I went back to *"Everyone has to die. What's the big deal?"* The "big deal" was the sudden imposition of a time frame and the choices that went along with that. Choices that affected not only me but those around me as well. Choices that were apparently mine and mine alone to make.

One choice I had made in the last year was to "whistle in the wind"—to while away my time *not* doing the things I knew I should be doing. Things that mattered. Like finishing my two novels. Like nurturing and loving and caring. I had wasted way too much of my time doing innane things until I finally realized that I had no time to waste. Every day must count. Each day, something must be accomplished. If not writing a chapter or two or three, then a bit of fun and joy.

MOUNTING FRUSTRATION

The mounting frustration of that last week in August was evident in my email exchange with Dr. Evans about getting my pathology samples to MDACC.

Hello Dr. Evans:

My slides were delivered this morning to "receiving" at MDACC. I have no idea if my MDACC patient number actually got properly associated with the slides. So, I hope they find their way to the right place.

The block uncut tumor did NOT go with the slides. Someone told me that a physician at MDACC must specifically request the block be sent.

The surgeon told me yesterday that the tumor board discussed my case yesterday and UH was going to do Epidermal Growth Factor Receptor (EGFR) mutation testing but, when I mentioned sending the slides to MDACC, he indicated that they would then NOT do the

EGFR testing and would see me when I "got back from Texas."

As you can imagine, my frustration (and fear) level has escalated substantially through all this. From my admittedly lay perspective, it appears to me that I need to get going on a course of treatment and that whoever is going to help determine that treatment needs as much information as possible. That information should include the EGFR mutation status of the BAC and perhaps even the meso, should it not?

If so, what should I do to expedite that testing? Should I strive to have it done before I see Dr. Fossella [professor and thoracic oncologist at MDACC] on Sept. 5?

Joann

Bless Dr. Evans for sending a reassuring reply.

Joann,

Anyone would be overwhelmed trying to deal with both your new diagnoses and the bureaucracy of the medical system. Try not to let it frustrate you any more than it has already. I'd rather you focus your energies on things like getting here safely, healing your thoracoscopy wounds, etc. It seems that we aren't going to have the EGFR data in hand next week, no matter what. Dr. Fossella assures me he can devise a plan, then amend it when that data become available, if necessary. Further, he copied me on his requests to our pathologists that this analysis be initiated on arrival.

We'll get the information. It'll affect only one drug in your potential plan, and we can add that drug slightly later, if necessary. I believe that University Hospital will send the block, hopefully it has already left. Either way, let's just follow up early next week, if we haven't already heard about it.

MANY people are aware of your case, and we're all looking forward to seeing you through this.

Scott Evans

Seeing me through what? My death seemed to be the only anticipated outcome. I didn't ask.

I was completely frustrated over trying to get the pathology samples from Colorado to Texas, something that seemed a straightforward task to me. I had emailed everyone even remotely involved at both University Hospital and MD Anderson on August 30.

Hello:

I checked with UH this morning. Despite the surgeon's email saying it was up to me whether or not to send the block to MDACC and despite my response email asking that it be sent, it was held up at UH because "they" wanted to take more pictures.

I've been assured that it will be sent to MDACC today. I hope this will be done. I presume it will be addressed to Dr. Kurie. I further presume that I'll be informed when it arrives tomorrow.

So, best case, the block will arrive on the Friday before Labor Day weekend. I'm assuming this means there will be no mutation information available before my appointment there on September 5.

To say that I am discouraged and disappointed is an understatement. Tomorrow will be three weeks since my biopsy. Before the surgery, the physicians involved all acknowledged that they were "aware of my wishes" vis-à-vis getting information to MDACC. Apparently, awareness does not translate to action.

The only positive spin I can possibly find in this is that perhaps UH actually started the EGFR genetic mutation testing and, if so, might actually share their results with you.

As my requests clearly have no effect, perhaps you could find out if they, in fact, have started the mutation testing.

Joann

GOING BACK TO HOUSTON

What a difference a year made. By Labor Day weekend in 2007, twelve months after the preliminary scan at National Jewish, I was en route to Houston with a double-death sentence diagnosis. Mesothelioma and unresectable BAC. How could this be? How was this possible? The two supposedly best institutions in the country had been watching my lungs and saying things like "benign etiology" and "probably inflammation." They even waited when a new spot showed up in my right lung and called that "probably inflammation." I just didn't get it!

I wrote a long email to Dr. Evans, essentially asking whether there was any hope for a few more years of life. I had written and sent it the night before, but by lunchtime Houston-time, there was still no response, even though he usually responded immediately to my emails.

So now I was doubly depressed. Of course, I was hoping he would say something like, "We caught it early, it's treatable, we can manage it," or *something* that would make it worthwhile to drive a thousand miles and use up a week or more of my apparently short remaining life. I was feeling like the trip to MD Anderson was a complete waste of time. Time that, at that moment, was very valuable to me.

So I took half a Valium. That helped for only a few hours. Then the knot in my stomach and the "almost tears" returned. Tears? Why? Frustration? Fear? Despair? Who knows? Sure, everyone has to die. But it's horrible to be faced with the reality. In-your-face reality, actually. Well, it was a chance to plan my own funeral, right? One final, great Joann party. I wondered what would happen at my funeral and sort of wished I could be there. Well, maybe I could at least plan it.

We began our long drive to Houston and I checked my email along the way. Correspondence with Dr. Evans continued over the issue of mutation testing and University Hospital's apparent reluctance to cooperate with MD Anderson in sharing either information or tumor samples. From somewhere in Oklahoma, I expressed my concerns to Dr. Evans.

On the subject of my case. I'm trying to assume that the meso is early stage but I have never succeeded in getting the surgeon (who is the only one who has actually seen my chest wall) to tell me much.

For example, I asked him how many lesions there were. He said "more than two." When I pressed my question, he said he didn't count them. When I asked about the possible risk of seeding more tumors from the unbagged biopsy, he answered, "That has never been proven."

I'm wondering if he has information that matters and, since this was VATS, does that mean there is a video (or photographs) that might be useful for you to have?

Joann

He replied:

Joann,

Answer 1: VATS procedures can be recorded, but since large video clips consume tons of memory, they aren't routinely. Short video clips and still images are fairly common, but purely discretionary to the person performing the procedure. So, I don't know if images were collected. His replies to your question suggest he wasn't likely to feel the need.

Answer 2: I don't think the number of lesions is likely to dramatically affect your treatment course. I suspect that an extrapleural pneu-monectomy is not likely, so your treatment is likely to be the same, regardless of the number of lesions.

Answer 3: He's right, there's no good data regarding seeding by biopsy. Probably a problem in certain liver and testicular can-cers, but mesothelioma is not established.

Scott Evans

ROTARY HOUSE IN HOUSTON

We arrived in Houston before Labor Day and checked into Rotary House. I managed to waste most of the first day, even though I knew I might regret it. I tried to tell myself that when I have a healthy day I need to use it wisely. Either back to writing the manuscript for my second mystery novel, *See How They Shine*, or, if I really couldn't focus, going to the office downstairs at Rotary to start printing email correspondence to and from doctors I had seen over the last fifteen months. That day, I really couldn't focus, so I printed emails. Later, I reworked a few chapters of the novel. I was up to chapter nine, but I hadn't even started the really hard stuff yet.

I felt a pain in my chest and the same old pain in my back and thought, *Are these symptoms?* Aargh.

> If you are unsure how long you will be treated, make a reservation for a longer time and then cancel. Not nice, but you certainly don't need more hassle.

I heard from a good friend and fellow cancer patient who had taken Carboplatin, used to treat cancers of the lungs. She reported that "it melted the tumors away like dry ice." That was great news. If only I would be able to send similar emails.

Because it took longer than we expected to get all of the tests scheduled at MDACC, we asked for an extension to our stay at Rotary House. They said no. Apparently, we weren't the only ones with housing problems. Roger overheard a woman on a cell phone near hysteria because they didn't have room for her at Rotary and she didn't know what to do. Not sure if she was trying to check in and they didn't have room or if she was being thrown out, as we were.

About eight that evening, the powers-that-be at Rotary decided we could stay one more night. Somehow, this business of not knowing whether we had a room was the proverbial straw that broke the camel's back. Why couldn't they do better at this? The Rotary card said, "The hotel with a heart." I wasn't so sure about that. I made a mental note that if we had to come back, I would make a reservation for a month and then leave early—when *we* were done, instead of going through that hassle again.

MAKING A PLAN

Given my prognosis, I thought that trip might well be my last to MD Anderson. After twenty-seven years of going there annually for follow-up visits after my breast cancer treatment in 1980, it felt really weird to think of never coming back.

That night, after attending the meditation program for patients, I logged on to MD Anderson's website to confirm that I still had an appointment with the Thoracic Center the next day. It turned out I was also scheduled for an appointment to do a PET/CT scan from skull to mid-thigh on September 20, two and half weeks away. That meant a total of twenty days in Houston at about $300 per day. *Not happening*, I thought. *We need to get out of Houston on Wednesday morning.*

I made a list of questions for my meeting the following day with my MDACC oncologist, Dr. Frank Fossella, paramount among them getting squared away with doing most of any ongoing treatment in Colorado. But first I needed to be clear on what "ongoing treatment" was . . . what the treatment plan was, how it would progress, and how we would keep up on progress. I had hopes that it all would shake down into a nice, neat clear plan and that I could get the records and slides that Dr. Mark Sitarik, my oncologist in Colorado, would want.

MY OWN PROFESSIONAL AND PERSONAL DEADLINES

The sense of urgency about keeping the original deadline for leaving Houston as planned was important to me professionally. I had secured one of eight coveted spots in a half-day workshop at the Rocky Mountain Fiction Writers (RMFW) three-day annual Colorado Gold writers conference, a proven place to meet editors and agents. I certainly didn't want to miss the opportunity since I had the manuscript of my first mystery for sale. I imagined that Roger could nap in the hotel room while I "performed" at the workshop in Denver.

Then I thought about the fun week going to the opera in San Francisco that was also in my near future plans. Opera had long been my passion. I love the spectacle, the beauty of the venues, the glory of the music—however silly the story.

I had recently learned how to let eBay know what things I might be interested in bidding on, and I put in "prepaid opera trips." Weeks later, whilst researching the dismal information on various cancers on the Internet, I got a chirpy note from eBay asking whether I might be interested in bidding on a week at the Inn at the Opera in San Francisco (not exactly a prepaid opera trip, but eBay's search function isn't perfect). *Why not?* I thought, and made a bid. A few days later, eBay sent me an email telling me that I had just "won" a 2-bedroom/2-bath furnished apartment at the Inn at the Opera from September 18 to 24, for $700.

Mentally, I walked through my schedule: MD Anderson wanted me in Houston until at least September 20. Before that, I was due at the RMFW workshop in Denver on Friday, September 14. *And* I had opera tickets in San Francisco on September 22 and 23. I weighed my options: If I skipped the writers' conference, I could get the PET/CT scan on September 20 in Houston, fly to San Francisco on the 21st, do the operas on the 22nd and the 23rd, and fly back to Houston on the 24th. Maybe my California friend and opera-going buddy could use the eBay apartment the 18th to the 20th.

But the workshop at the writers' conference offered a half-day to meet with an acquisitions editor. A half-day when he would focus on only eight manuscripts. I felt I really should not miss that opportunity. Why couldn't I get the PET/CT scan at home in Boulder? The short answer, of course, was because MD Anderson did all the other scans, so the previous results were readily available for comparison. Comparison by the same institution is a plus, just as comparison over time is a plus.

Totally conflicted about what to do, I expanded my focus from where to have further tests to what else might need to be done. I bugged the ever-patient Dr. Evans about my continuing concern that the mesothelioma had been spread along the removal tract during the biopsy. I had read a lot about excruciating results of such tumor seeding that can be alleviated by immediate X-ray therapy.

Hello:

Thank you for your patience in answering.

Re: radiation. My first response is Aarggh. My second response is I think I should do it somewhere. This is a gut feeling probably fueled by a latent distrust of the surgeon, which I realize is rationally unreasonable, but . . .

I don't see how I could get it done in Boulder before September 25, which is 47 days post-surgery. Is that too late? (Probably you don't know the answer to that.) And it might even be longer than that, given that I'd have to get it set up somehow.

So, maybe a one-shot deal here [MDACC] would be best IF it could be done this week. Can you see if that's in any realm of likeli-hood?

Joann

His response was a reassuring one.

Joann:

It is both a genuine pleasure and a bona fide challenge of academic medicine to work with

patients who are sufficiently sophisticated as to identify latent distrust in themselves as a motivating factor.

I heard back from Dr. Fossella this morning. He recommends against the radiation. Recognizing my role as your advocate relative to his role as your primary treating oncologist, my recommendation is that you meet with him to discuss this directly (even though the wait for an overbook spot may be frustratingly long). The weakness of the available literature suggests that neither of you can make an irrefutable case for or against the intervention. He seems to have been sufficiently open to your suggestions to facilitate your (subsequently aborted) surgical evaluation. I see no reason why he wouldn't be similarly available for a discussion with you now.

I recognize that you have many factors driving you to want to do something immediately. Systemic chemotherapy alone may be the best "something" you can do right now. I'd allow Dr. Fossella to present his arguments against radiation.

Scott Evans

After a final meeting with Dr. Fossella, we decided to proceed in Boulder with chemotherapy, which, in his words, "might let you live two years or so." We prepared to decamp Houston on September 5 during a brewing hurricane. Humberto, soon downgraded to a tropical storm, was just one more thing to deal with at that point.

I sent an email to Jon Kurie, the researcher with MD Anderson who got me into the thoracic appointment process in a timely manner and about whose work I have written occasionally over the years.

> *Subject: leaving tomorrow*
>
> *Hi Jon:*
>
> *I saw Dr. Fossella today and he said you had asked about me.*
>
> *Basically, I gather there is little to be done. I'm going to try Alimta and Carboplatin (and maybe something else depending on the EGFR results, which are still pending). If they don't work, as Dr. Fossella said, "We're right back where we are now." Which seems to be not much of anywhere.*
>
> *It's a very weird feeling, after 27 years of coming to MDACC, to suddenly be so "at sea." It's also quite surreal after all the watchful waiting of the last 14 months, which entailed various people telling me they were*

watching carefully in order to catch anything bad "early."

It seems, at least from my present perspective, as though what we've done with this "early" diagnosis is give me more time for psychological distress. (When I'm in a better frame of mind, I do try to see the situation as "more time for getting things finished up.")

Nonetheless, I certainly thank you for your help in getting me this timely consult. I do like Dr. Fossella a lot. Just wish he had some even quasi-magic bullet.

His parting remark this afternoon was to let him hear from me with "good news." I'd like to think that's possible.

Joann

Jon responded empathetically:

Joann

I wish we did have a magic bullet. The agents Frank proposes to use are effective in some people. Let's hope for the best.

Jon

CHAPTER THREE

THE START OF GOLD STANDARD TREATMENT

O n Friday, September 14, 2007, we were back in Denver and checked into the Renaissance Hotel for the Rocky Mountain Fiction Writers annual conference. We had first stopped in Boulder instead of going directly to the workshop at the writers' conference in Denver so I could have a B-12 shot, which I needed before I could start chemo. I had the shot on Friday because the doctor wasn't going to be in on Monday, a date I would have preferred since getting the shot on Monday meant I wouldn't miss any part of the three-day conference. I had learned last minute while traveling through Kansas on our way home that I would have to get the shot on Friday, and spent quite a bit of time arguing on the phone with a number of people about whether I could get the shot before or after the conference.

But as we crossed the Colorado border, I gave up, agreed to come back to Boulder on Friday and miss the eight-person-only half-day workshop. (Of course, when I got to Boulder, I got the shot, and didn't even have to see the doctor after all.) Back at the conference the next day, I was nearly late for a ten-minute pitch appointment with the acquisitions editor from Five Star whose workshop I had missed the day before.

The editor spent one of my allotted ten minutes observing, "No one ever missed a workshop with me before," and then spent another two minutes or so telling me why he didn't like my story (*See How They Scurry*). But then he said he loved my writing and asked whether I had anything else. I told him about *See How They Shine*. He said, "Tell me the story." I did. He asked, "Same characters?" Yes. "Including the dog?" Again, yes. Finally, he said, "Okay, can you send me the whole manuscript in the next four weeks?" *Yes!*

Then I went up to the room and cried for an hour. Roger thought I had totally lost my mind. Could I send the editor my manuscript in four weeks? How the Sam Hill did I know? It wasn't quite done; actually, it was done except for the last chapter, but it also really needed rewriting. For sure it was going to be a mess to format because most of it was in individual chapters, and word processing is far from my finest skill.

Disjointed thoughts displaced planning. I was leaving for San Francisco in forty-eight hours. I surmised, *Maybe I could rewrite the blasted manuscript in my apartment at the Inn at the Opera.* Then I was supposed to start chemo on September 26. *Could I work on the book then?*

ON THE CANCER SIDE OF THINGS

On the cancer side of things, many people were trying to help. Randi Londer Gould, a former student of mine, who had become a good friend and was now managing editor of an oncology journal, asked the physician who was director of both the Albert Einstein College of Medicine and the Cancer Centers at Beth Israel Medical Center in New York to try to help. An email from him was waiting for me when we returned to Boulder on Sunday. He was checking up on me and asking, "Are you home yet? Can I call you?" I had to smile.

Steve Schneider, author of *The Patient from Hell*, was a friend and fellow cancer patient who had chronicled his own experiences in cancer treatment. He had sent me emails pointing out that he "walked away from his own funeral" by "going offshore." Roger and I had found some promising work on meso in Europe, which is where Steve had gone for his rare, dreadful disease treatment. It was nice to know people were thinking about my problem.

AN OPERATIC REPRIEVE

Only two operas were scheduled while I was in San Francisco for my eBay trip, but I was willing to see both. So I had tickets to Saint-Saëns' *Samson and Delilah* and

Wagner's *Tännhauser*. One small problem with the trip to San Francisco was that Roger hates opera. But that was easily solved by enticing a friend to come up from her home in Sunnyvale to spend some time with me and go to one opera. She went to *Samson and Delilah,* and either enjoyed or endured it—a bit of both probably. It rained on and off only one day that week, and that was the day we had planned to spend at Japantown, which is mostly inside, so even that worked out well. We went to the Asian Art Museum, heard Wangari Maathai (Kenyan environmental and political activist) speak at Herbst, and attended the Target Family Concert of the San Francisco Symphony.

The latter was truly remarkable. Target gave this concert as a gift to the children of San Francisco. The audience was at least 30% under age 10 and some much younger. Tickets were $10 each for any seat in the house. Target also provided entertainment and free snacks beforehand. The bars were piled high with cartons of milk, veggie cups, and fruit kabobs. After the concert, there were balloons and fortune cookies—the universal fortune: "Music Brings Families Together."

The beauty of all of the above is that all these amazingly fun events were within two blocks of the Inn at the Opera, so no worries about getting "home" afterwards. On one trip home, we cut through the side courtyard of the opera. There we encountered an interesting group outside the stage door: a white horse, a handler, and a man in a magenta, swoopy sort of costume. Said man was talking to the horse in a very basso-profundo voice, saying something to the effect of "How you doing, old boy?" We marveled a bit at the horse, petted it after receiving permission from the handler, and went on our way. Several nights later, when I saw *Tännhauser*, the horse and the magenta-clad man made their spectacular entrance at the end of Act I. He was one of the principals of the opera. I hope it didn't hurt his ego that these ditzy women were talking to the horse and ignoring him in the courtyard on opening night.

Mid-trip, the "opera duty" went to another California friend who not only likes opera but was willing to see *Tännhauser*. (Wagner can go on and on and on, but *Tännhauser* was really interesting.) David Gockley, newly in San Francisco from Houston, made his mark with the staging for this opera. Very, very like the Houston Grand Opera, and not much like the usual San Francisco Opera. Venus ran around in a sheet for four hours, made her last entrance in full voice lolling across the backs of four crawling, mostly naked guys, and the stage had fire effects three or four times. The next day, the newspaper review said something to the effect of "fire came often and stayed too long." I agreed with that. The reviewer also called the horse "gratuitous," but that's because he hadn't met him up close and personal. He was *not* gratuitous, he was just uneasy—and who wouldn't be with all those trumpets and guys storming around waving swords and so forth, not to mention an entire chorus dressed in blue drapes and gold crowns. (This was an in-your-face reference to the Virgin

Mary, just in case anyone missed the distinction between Venus loosely wrapped in a sheet and the heroine Elizabeth who sacrificed herself to go to heaven to plead directly for the redemption of Tännhauser. The effect was only slightly marred by the typo in the supertitles referring to the Virgin May).

Even my trip home from San Francisco was interesting. I got to the airport early. Two metal knees makes going through security a sometimes quite lengthy process. I had lunch at a sit-down food court, and a couple who were quite chatty joined me. They introduced themselves as having a "born again conservative" background. They were en route to his mother's funeral, but, as he said, he wasn't distressed because he knew his mother was now at peace with Jesus. I thought, *It sure would be nice to have such certainty.* I told my tablemates the story of Tännhauser (more or less). While they seemed unfamiliar with opera in general, they were quite pleased to learn that everybody was eligible for redemption—except, of course, the ladies running around in sheets.

It turned out that my award ticket home was in first class on a 777. I'd never been on one of those before. First class is so big it has two bathrooms. The seats are nice, roomy, have foot rests, *and* I played with my new iPod all the way home. I sent blessings to the friend who gave me the iPod for my birthday and had secretly skimmed CDs out of our house and downloaded my faves onto it. I was deep into listening to *Carmina Burana* with Kathleen

Battle when I realized we had landed at DIA. Good earphones helped me to miss all the stuff about putting your tray tables in their "upright and locked positions" and so forth.

DAY ONE OF CHEMO

I returned home from San Francisco on my 69th birthday, September 24, 2007. A deluge of birthday cards were waiting for me, thanks to the prompting of a friend. I spent a lot of time with these cards and the fond thoughts of the people who sent them.

My first day of chemo, two days later, was a much more gentle experience than it had been in 1980. Nice cushy recliners, refreshments, TVs with earphones so you listen only if you want to, and lots of folks responding to your needs. But it also involved the same scary drugs and the same unsettling mix of inconsistent information.

I actually was supposed to start chemo the day before, but Rocky Mountain Cancer Center (RMCC) in Boulder, where I was receiving my treatments, was *out* of the Alimta. It occurred to me to wonder why. Maybe they don't use it very often. Maybe that was a potential problem, but maybe it wasn't.

I looked up the pharmaceutical information on Alimta on the web and discovered that in addition to the B-12 shot and the folic acid I had in the ten days before chemo, I was also supposed to have taken a steroid twice on the day before chemo. This was to be followed by doses the day of chemo and the day after chemo. The steroid is specifically taken to deter a rash that often occurred during treatment with Alimta. My last brush with chemo, twenty-seven years before, had produced a leprosy-like look for many weeks. I was not eager to repeat that.

I took a copy of the web printout and gave it to the nurse at RMCC. He went off to talk to the doctor and eventually came back and said, "It's okay because we're giving you 10 mg of steroid in the initial drip, but we'll call in a script for the rest of it." *A steroid in the initial drip isn't exactly the same thing as the day before*, I thought. *But did it really matter?*

Treatment started with the initial drip, consisting of the steroid and a mild sedative. Next was the Alimta, which is supposed to be "pushed" in over the course of ten minutes instead of dripping slowly. The head nurse, who started the Alimta push, told me, "We will wait at least thirty minutes after this finishes before starting the Carboplatin." I failed to ask why, but in retrospect, I should have.

There was only a short break after the Alimta was done and as I was settling in, the nurse began to fiddle with the IV bags. "Did you start the Carboplatin?" I asked. She had. "I think you're supposed to wait thirty minutes," I said, not very calmly. She switched it off and went away. In the meantime, my IV line filled up to the clamp with blood. When she came back, she had another huge bag of saline with her. "We'll just drip saline for half an hour," she said, "then I'll start the Carboplatin." No mention of why, and sounding a little as if the whole thing had been her idea in the first place.

I didn't know whether it really mattered; that is, whether waiting thirty minutes was important or not. I grumbled to myself: I just hate it when people tell me different things and I don't know which is right, and I have a funny feeling that it might matter—maybe even matter a whole lot.

While I waited, the guy across the aisle from me started up a conversation. It turned out that he had been observing the above interaction while pretending to read his book. His opening line to me: "Didn't you used to work at the Department of Commerce?" Surprised, I said, "Yes, I did." After a more lengthy conversation, he revealed that, at an American Geophysical Union meeting in San Francisco sometime around 1976, I had been "really annoyed" with him in a press conference. I, of course, had no memory of this, but I must have been really impressive because later he said to the young woman who came back to start the Carboplatin, "You really don't want her pissed off at you."

Thirty years. Either he has a very good memory or I was in very fine form that day. Either way, he decided I didn't recognize him because he had no hair. Okay. Maybe, maybe not. Then his wife showed up. She was a chemistry teacher and didn't have any bones to pick with me, so we had a nice conversation.

The parting confusion came back to the steroid. Roger had picked up the prescription while I was sitting in a chair being "pampered," in a chemo sort of way. The label on the bottle read, "Take two pills on days 1 through 5 of chemo." Now, this was not taking the steroid only the aforementioned three times, the day before, the day of, and the day after chemo, which is what Eli Lilly's Alitma website said to do. Furthermore, I had just gotten 10 mg of it in a drip.

When I first read these directions, we had already left the chemo infusion area, saying "See you tomorrow" to the folks there on our way out. We decided to go back to question the dosage. The first person I encountered was a nice young woman, who said with a wry smile, "Wow, is it tomorrow already?"

I told her I needed clarification about the steroid and explained what I'd read and what the directions said to do. She went away and came back with the instruction that I should take just one that evening (4 mg) because the 10 mg in the drip would count as the first day's dose.

This still didn't address the "day before" issue for the next round of chemo, but I figured I had twenty days to find out about that. So, on day one I had 14 mg of steroid and then 8 mg on each of the next four days. Then I was supposed to just stop. This, I feared, could make me crazy on the day I did stop. (Fortunately, it didn't.)

SOME NEEDED ALONE TIME

The next day, I felt an overwhelming need to be alone—away from the phone, away from people—just alone. I drove the short distance to Veterans Park, a little-used park above Valmont Lakes, where the view of Boulder Valley and the mountains beyond is filtered by the smokestacks of a local power plant.

There were two other cars there, both parked to enjoy the west-facing view of the mountains. So I parked on the side of the lot looking south. This provided an unexpected view: shrubs, bushes, fir trees, and leafless—perhaps even dead—deciduous trees, which filled both sides of Arapahoe Road. Behind them, atop the hill, was our house. It was the only house visible. The dead trees, stark in the landscape between me and my home, reminded me of the desolation of Wagner's *Venusberg*. I pondered, *Will they, too, burst into flame?* Surely not.

I watched our house for a while and wondered, *Will death be like that? Seeing but not connected? Near, but yet so far?*

Later that day, I reported back to Rocky Mountain Cancer Center for a Neulasta shot. All $6200 of it. This drug, heavily advertised, claimed to boost the white blood count, thus offering protection from opportunistic infections. To me, it was just more drugs.

TAKING MEASURES INTO MY OWN HANDS

There was still much to do. The most important: figuring out how to get into remission and stay there. I started seriously thinking about how to collect, understand, organize, and assess information on mesothelioma. Mesothelioma is an orphan disease, meaning it is so rare that no one is researching treatments. Rocky Mountain Cancer Center had had only one other meso patient, and my Boulder oncologist, Dr. Sitarik, had treated only one other meso patient in his career. Alimta, one of the chemo drugs I was receiving, was "standard of care" for meso, but a "standard" that staved off death by maybe a few months, if it worked at all.

Since we were dealing with two uniformly fatal cancers, the treatment plan at that time appeared to be some variant of: First, per the Hippocratic Oath, do no harm and try "standard care." Then, when "standard care" quits working or doesn't work, wait for symptoms to develop. Treat those symptoms and spare the patient pain until her inevitable death.

This hardly seemed like a "treatment" plan, and I wasn't willing to go along with it. There had to be something better. I set out to find it. Concurrent with this search for effective treatment, I attempted to grasp what sanity I could.

The beginning of October 2007, one week after my first chemo, I went to a meeting of the Boulder Chapter of Sisters in Crime (SinC), a national professional organization of mystery writers. They helped me with a professional problem brought about by my unexpected cancer diagnosis. After several years of submitting my first mystery fiction manuscript to various possible publishers, I had finally gotten a firm nibble. An editor for a mainline publisher was interested. Interested enough to read the entire manuscript and make very concrete suggestions for a straightforward rewrite.

I celebrated when I got the letter and then, after accepting her proposal for a rewrite, set to work on it. Then I had some second thoughts. If they accepted my rewrite, they would purchase my manuscript for an advance against royalties. They would then own the manuscript. They could publish it immediately, or in six or eighteen months, or maybe even never. Further, they would demand right of first refusal on any subsequent manuscripts using the same characters.

I had finished the second manuscript in the series and was preparing to start on the third. Under normal circumstances, I would have welcomed this standard newbie contract. But I was not in normal circumstances. If I accepted it, I might not live long enough to see my books in print. What to do?

Self-publishing was beginning to flourish. But it was still certainly looked down on as a venue where those with no other options frequently took their ill-written tomes.

Would self-publishing affect sales of my book? Probably, but newbies don't get a lot of marketing help from their publishers these days anyway. Would self-publishing affect the look of my book? Not if I could make all the parts come together: cover art, testimonials from other mystery authors, bio, author photo, solid editing, infallible proofreading, an enticing webpage, and seemingly always one more thing. One more thing that I had never done before. It was difficult and at least one typo snuck through. (But, as I tell myself gleefully, so do typos sneak through in hardback, mainline fiction. Not often, but they are there.)

The SinC group helped me crystallize my feelings and I decided to go the self-publishing route. After that lengthy discussion, a dear friend in the group presented me with a beautiful white silk scarf that had been blessed by the Dalai Lama's monks in Tibet. She told the tale of first climbing hundreds of steps at a daunting 12,000-foot altitude to reach the Potala Palace, where she intended to have the scarf blessed, only to learn the monks were not in residence. She then traveled to the Jokhang Temple, considered to be one of the most sacred and important of the Buddhist temples, where the scarf was blessed. I certainly appreciated her beautiful and humbling gesture.

GETTING OUT MORE

A few days later, I was able to go church with a "DO NOT HUG" sign that a friend had made for me to keep potentially germy folks away. Everyone was very amused. The featured speaker talked about how the God of Jesus was the God of the Jews, that the Kingdom of God was "here and now" and evident in the way we live with and treat each other. A very powerful sermon for where I was at that moment.

These had been big days for me: church, concerts, professional meetings, and rehab time in the pool. I felt really good except for an occasional *wham-o* pain in my lower back. More than likely the pain was the Neulasta shot I had a few days before, jacking around with my bone marrow and firing it up to boost my white blood cells.

Later that week, I went to a meeting of my church group, New Women, where I shared what I had written in response to an exercise called "This I Believe" (www.thisibelieve.org):

I believe in connections. Connections with people. Connections with the past. Connections with the future. Connections nurture me, sustain me. empower me.

I enjoy things that remind me of connections. For example, soft, well-worn handkerchiefs left over from childhood. The comfort of a small, green hankie with black and white bulldogs on it is hard to replicate. I use my little green hankie a lot more lately. And appreciate it more as well.

I believe that everywhere is somewhere. This belief hits the wall at the scale of the universe. Where is the universe? If everything is somewhere, then the universe must be somewhere also. But . . .

I don't have the same stonewall feeling on the other end of the spectrum. Should have, I suppose, but it seems easier to keep thinking smaller and smaller then it is to keep thinking larger and larger.

I wished I knew what I believed about anything else.

I had experienced a fair amount of pain in the morning before that meeting, seemingly in my left lung. I wondered, *Can I hope that this is the chemo eating the tumor? Does that hurt?* A nice thought, but it probably wasn't true.

That day, a cousin called from Illinois with the news that her daughter was getting married in October of next year. My first thought was, *I hope I'm alive to go.*

SECOND CYCLE OF CHEMO

My second cycle of chemo began three weeks later, at the end of October. Shortly thereafter, I had a most encouraging talk with Dr. Sitarik. He said he had been thinking about me while driving to work that day, and he agreed that we needed to be looking beyond "standard care." He mentioned the possibility of doing an assay of living tissue, which would measure the functionality of the chemo treatment I was receiving. It was really the only way to get a handle on the genetic or molecular basis of my cancers. This, of course, would require more surgery, but he went on to say that he hoped, with creative use of CT and PET technology, to be able to identify a "two-fer" and get sufficient tissue samples from both cancers to allow an assay without yet another surgical biopsy. I hoped so, but rather doubted it. (My skepticism was rooted in the fact that no one could see the meso on any noninvasive test for more than a year, so why would this time be any different?)

Dr. Sitarik also said that if Neulasta had worked the first time, it would continue to work, so I wouldn't have to be quite so worried about catching bugs, to which he added, "But it *is* flu season, remember." What was that about "the right hand giveth while the left hand taketh away"?

When I first got settled in the chemo room, one of my "colleagues" there thought to entertain me with tales of how his second Neulasta shot had caused a lot of bone pain, and someone else chimed in to be sure that I knew that it got worse with each shot. The conversation concluded with an encouraging thought from one of these fellow patients: "It felt like a vulture was trying to claw my breastbone out." Jeez! Count that among the things I did not need to know. At that point, it seemed best to stick the iPod earbuds in my ears, close my eyes, and listen to *O Fortuna*.

I felt fine going into chemo, and I felt mostly okay later that day. After the last round of chemo treatments, I had been pretty much okay until three or four days after each treatment. But this time I felt well enough to plan on going to some concerts at the College of Music, where we had gone to a vibraphone concert earlier that week.

"MANAGING" MY DOCTORS

Dr. Sitarik had asked me to email my questions in advance of our next meeting, scheduled for October 31, so he could have time to think about them. I began the challenging task of distilling my hundreds of questions into a reasonable number and a manageable format.

> *Hi, Dr. Sitarik:*
>
> *This sort of mushroomed . . . but, attached is my list of questions plus some narrative as to why I'm asking these questions.*

See you on Halloween!

Joann

To this short email, I attached the following questions. Dr. Sitarik did not answer those questions marked by an asterisk. Comments made by me in retrospect, months later, are indicated in square brackets.

Attachment: Questions for Dr. Sitarik

My questions seem to fall into three categories. I'll call them philosophy, options, and facts. My questions are listed immediately below. Following the question list is a bit of discourse that should explain why I'm asking these questions. I've keyed the discourse to the questions.

PHILOSOPHY

1. Do you and I agree on the goal of my treatment?

2. What is your likely expectation for progression?

3. Does it matter what I eat? (For example, is sugar pouring gas on the cancer fire?)

OPTIONS

1.   Am I going to get genetic profiling? Or some attempt to individualize targeted therapy? Drug selection?

2.   Should we continue the present chemo regime? (Said another way: How will I know if you think the Carboplatin is being effective?)

3.   Can we add a VEGF [(vascular endothelial growth factor] inhibitor to my regime now?

4*. Should we add the antidepressant desipramine?

5*. Should we switch from Zocor to lovastatin?

6*. Is there any other drug with synergistic effect on chemo (e.g., indibulin)?

FACTS

1.   Do I have effusions?

2.   Do I have distant mets?

3.   Do I have positive nodes?

4.   Are there any circumstances under which I'm a candidate for BAC resection? [This would turn out, nearly a year later, to be a prophetic question.]

5. Are there any circumstances under which I'm a candidate for meso debulking surgery?

6*. Is my BAC nonmucinous/mucinous/ mixed?

7. We're assuming the GGOs in my right lung are BAC. Could this be wrong? [Yes, we were wrong, but we didn't find this out until September 2008.]

8. What is my tumor load?

Philosophy, Question 1

As I understand the goal of my tx [treatment], it cannot be curative. While my long-range goal doubtless harbors hope of a "fix," I would state my present goal as: to live as long as possible, as comfortably and productively as possible.

Philosophy, Question 2

When pressed for a prognosis, Dr. Fossella said I "might live several years." My first reading of the dismal literature on both BAC and meso, made "several years" seem an unlikely hope; however, recent results do seem to be more hopeful. [Hillerdal, G., et al. International Association for the Study of Lung Cancer meeting, Sept. 2007: 44% survival/

18 months. Like all recent "good news" reports about meso, the regimen included some sort of targeted tx (gemcitabine in this case).]

Van den Bogaert et al. (Jour Thor Ono 1, 1, January 2006, p.25-30) appears to say that maintenance tx with Alimta changes median survival from 6 to 14.7 months. This was after 6 cycles of Alimta/Carboplatin and total 8-20 additional Alimta tx. (Table 2, p. 29). Authors say: "threefold longer TTO and OS . . . especially remarkable because 5 of 13 in the maintenance group already relapsed after first-line tx."

Options, Question 1

If it is not clear which VEGF inhibitor to use, should we try to individualize this with gene expression profiling to describe these tumors well enough to select likely targets and/or drugs? If so, can we please get started on this process?

There seems to be no biologically-based method for selecting the best drug for a patient but there were a lot of new techniques discussed last week at the AACR-NCI-EORTC meeting in San Francisco. Would any of these work on the blocks in paraffin, which are available at UH?

Options, Question 3

Everything I have read shows a measurable benefit from adding targeted therapy. And much in the literature argues for concurrent treatment with chemo and targeted therapy (most recently, "Avastin with Chemo or Tarceva Superior to Chemo Alone in NSCLC," Herbst, R. et al., Journal Clin Onc, Oct 1, 2007, 12:3026).

Options, Question 4

At the AACR-NCI-EORTC meeting last week, Farrell et al. reported that desipramine (anti-depressant) "greatly augments the cytotoxicity of platinum-based chemo." The synergistic effect of desipramine resulted in increased activation of p53, mitochondrial damage, caspase activation, and PARP cleavage.

89% had some tumor shrinkage.

Options, Question 5

Same meeting as Q4: Trinh et al. B240 report lovastatin inhibits VEGFR function and induces synergistic cytotoxity in mesothelioma cells . . . in combination with VEGFR inhibitors. I am on Zocor. Presumably it would be okay to switch to lovastatin. Dosages may be much higher.

Options, Question 6

Same meeting as Q4: Abstract B276/targets microtubes.

Facts, all Questions

At the Seven Levels of Healing, Dr. Fleagle drew a flow chart of cancer tx.

bx → dx → stage → tx → evaluation of results.

*My questions relate to the **stage** and **evaluation** steps of this flow chart. First, for the meso. I don't know stage, grade, and I know very little about the extent of the disease. Here's what I do know. The pulmonologist at MDACC described it as "minimal." The UH surgeon said there was a "large mass" rising from the diaphragm and lesions on the chest wall. I asked him how many lesions. He said "more than two." I repeated my question and he said "I didn't count them."*

Second, for the BAC, I know it is Stage IV because it's in more than one lobe and probably more than one lung. (But we're assuming the right lung GGOs are the same thing and no "assumption" about any of this has yet been correct.) Dr. Fossella told me my Stage IV is not the "same thing" as a Stage IV with distant mets.

Facts, Question 5

I asked you about reducing the "large mass" on my diaphragm with Cyberknife. You said it wouldn't change the outcome. My question around that issue is: Since drugs have to get to the cells via blood flow, isn't it easier for the drugs to work on smaller tumors? So, why isn't it better to make tumors smaller, if possible?

Joann

Several months later, when I picked up copies of all the notes on my case to take to my cardiologist at University Hospital, I found that Dr. Sitarik complained about my four-page email. I guess the email *was* four pages, but it began as a *dozen* questions and 20 pages. In addition, he had included other complaints about the amount of his time I take. In an effort to take less time, I developed a new strategy. After every scan, I requested a copy of the scan and report before I saw Dr. Sitarik again. This gave me a chance to think about any questions the scan might raise.

On the subject of "too much time": appointments with my doctor were scheduled for *fifteen* minutes. During that time, the doctor was supposed to examine me, discuss any new findings, present any new plans and answer any questions. Fifteen minutes. Ha!

If you need more time, ask for it when you book your appointment.

CHEMO CYCLE NUMBER THREE

It would be nice to say that it was immediately obvious whether the chemo was working, or more accurately, *not* working. Not so. A CT scan was scheduled for the first week in November 2007, with round three of chemo tentatively scheduled to begin shortly thereafter, depending on the results of the scan. I didn't want to go ahead with chemo cycle number three without assurance that there was some reason to do so.

During the subsequent meeting with Dr. Sitarik, in addition to discussing my questions, he told me that the latest CT scan had shown that some of the lesions were smaller, which was encouraging. So it was a "go" for the next round of chemo.

Chemo treatment number three in the first half of November had more than its share of the usual hassles. Nothing went as it had before; therefore, I objected to just about every step in the process. The problem started the moment I arrived. The first thing they said to me was: "You're a week early." "Nope," I replied, "it's been three weeks." They confirmed that it had indeed been three weeks, but they had me scheduled for the following week. They would take me, yes, but everything seemed screwed up from then on.

To administer a round of chemo takes about two hours, and they won't start if they don't think they can be done by 5:00. When I finally got to the chemo room, it was 2:45 p.m. But the chemo wasn't ready. It hadn't been mixed because they hadn't expected me until the following week. A nurse I had never seen before showed up and stood in front of me, reading intently from a single sheet of paper she had in her hand. She said, "I guess we'll start with the Carboplatin, it's ready."

"That's not how it's been done in the past," I responded. My patience was wasting away as quickly as the time left to complete my treatment. "You started with the Alimta because it's an IV push, has a short half-life, and needs not to be fighting with anything else during its short and, as I just discovered, $17,465 half-life." To which she said, "No, it's okay to go with the Carboplatin first."

I muttered something to the effect of, "I can't decide right or wrong but it's different and I don't like it." She resorted to the old saw, "It's what your doctor ordered," which gave me my opening: "Show me his order, please."

Apparently, this was not the piece of paper she had in her hand because she went away and I never saw her again. Soon afterwards, the head nurse showed up with the Alimta and started it without further comment. I, of course, was completely freaked out by this time and commented further . . . much, much further.

I suppose I was just so close to the edge that I couldn't stand anything unexpected, but then again there's the very short—and very expensive—half-life of Alimta. The chemo was finished before 5:00 p.m., and mercifully a friend was waiting in the wings to take me home.

After the last chemo, my hemoglobin tanked, and, coupled with Boulder's 5,500-foot altitude, any semblance of energy or willingness to do anything completely disappeared. I lay around doing nothing. The fact that I was only halfway through this chemo regime was very off-putting, given the mental fog I waded through the week following the chemo. Taking a drug to combat the effects of another drug and then a third drug to combat the effects of the second was a "drug cascade" that just didn't seem like a good idea when I was rational enough to know what a good idea might be.

With Thanksgiving less than a week away, I tried to count my blessings.

> *I'm thankful to be alive at this point.*
> *I'm thankful that good friends will share*
> *Thanksgiving with us, and that someone else*
> *is doing almost all of the cooking. I'm very*
> *thankful for all my friends, who are helping in*
> *so many ways. And, thanks to a lot of re-*
> *search, emailing, and study by several*

dedicated researchers, the "powers that be" are looking at my tumor blocks for VEGF mutations with the thought of adding a targeted therapy.

I'm also thankful for the new, comprehensive Rocky Mountain Cancer Center here in Boulder. Roger and I have both used many of the "extras" they offer, including the cinnamon buns at the snack bar and a wealth of classes, talks, and demonstrations.

RMCC'S COMPLIMENTARY THERAPIES

Rocky Mountain Cancer Center really made the effort to reach out and be sure their patients knew about anything and everything that might be helpful. In addition, it had much complementary therapy to offer its patients. It was wonderful that RMCC was only seven minutes from our house.

The evening after my third chemo, Roger and I went back to RMCC for their drop-in musical therapy group. There was a great facilitator and new instruments: lots of different drums, wooden and metal xylophones, tambourines, cowrie bell gourds, and rain sticks.

The facilitator started the session by asking whether anybody wanted to say anything. I volunteered most of my

Among the talks offered by RMCC was a special talk by a representative of Share the Care (sharethecare.org), an online organization geared toward helping to organize care for people with all sorts of needs.

day's ordeal, and someone else said he had encountered a similar problem but had trouble "being present" enough to argue about it. He therefore spent the next week worrying whether his chemo had been compromised. At least I didn't have to worry about compromised chemo.

Then we picked out our instruments. I got a very big drum on which I banged enthusiastically, even if not very musically, for thirty to forty minutes while we were "playing." It was amazingly cathartic. The facilitator suggested that I might want to try a more "subtle" instrument. So I got a metallic xylophone, which still allowed me to make more noise than anyone else. I had a great time!

The next day, I tried acupuncture at RMCC. The therapist earned her master's degree at Oregon and then spent three years in China, where she trained and worked at two hospitals. She worked on opening energy channels to my eyes, hands, and feet, and after about an hour, I felt totally relaxed, happy, and simply marvelous. I thought, *this may just be working!* I went to see her again the following week. The acupuncture therapy really helped with both my distorted vision (a side effect of the chemo drugs) and my numb feet.

Roger and I also attended a Qigong (pronounced Chi-Gong) class, which was an introduction to Chinese energy healing. The practitioner took us through an hour's worth of energy enhancement, something I sorely needed.

Even better, the Center for Integrative Healing at RMCC had grape hard candies to suck on that did not taste like metal. Because of the chemo, everything else, especially water, tasted like really nasty metal. The suggestion given to me to avoid this gross assault on my taste buds was to use "strong flavors such as lemon or lime." Yuck. Lemon metal is lemon metal no matter what. Garlic worked, curry worked. and these fake, overwhelmingly grape-y hard candies apparently worked.

For those who were interested, there was a special presentation about "Looking Good While Haggard" (my version of the title—the actual title was a little more nuanced, "Look Good, Feel Better") that offered free wigs, makeup tips, and so on. My hair had managed to hang on the whole time, so instead of attending this presentation, I hoped to have the energy to be busy getting *See How They Scurry* whipped into publication shape. My goal was to have the rewrites finished before November 29, my next date with infused toxic platinum.

SPIRITUAL HEALING WORKSHOP

After Thanksgiving, I realized how uncomfortable I was with the "journey" concept so many people used to describe the cancer process. This metaphor was particularly prominent in the Seven Levels of Healing workshop, which extended over almost two months. To me, this had not been a journey through cancer. It had been a journey *imposed by* cancer with a fixed destination that was *inescapable.*

Getting to know the other patients in the Seven Levels of Healing group was tremendously valuable, and the social worker and oncology nurse who facilitated the workshop were exceptional. This workshop helped to lead to a time of spiritual healing. Among the things suggested for me to try was keeping a daily journal addressing the following questions:

1. How do I feel today? What emotions have I experienced in the last twenty-four hours?

2. How do I feel about my cancer? How is it impacting my life?

3. What am I willing to give up to heal or to overcome this cancer?

4. What are the gifts this cancer has brought/can bring to me and my family?

What the heck. I decided to give it the old college try. I started my journal on Sunday, December 7, 2007.

1.   Today I feel discouraged, scared, and despairful. Time is slipping by. I must get on with my writing, both this journal and See How They Shine. Yesterday, I was encouraged by stuff on the web from people with mesothelioma living long lives. Today I cannot find it. Only downer stuff.

2.   Cancer is running my life. Appointments here, there, everywhere. Are acupuncture and Healing Touch what I need? Yes. Also the gym, I think.

There was nothing for either point three or four because I couldn't think of anything other than wanting the cancer to heal and I certainly couldn't think of any gifts it had brought. Apparently, at that moment, this journaling wasn't working for me.

CHAPTER FOUR

A CHANGE IN THE COURSE OF MY TREATMENT

December 2007 brought with it my fourth chemo session, which proceeded smoothly without "fireworks," as a friend put it. No fireworks until the end, that is, when the bandage on my vein let go. The resulting bloody mess eventually "healed" into a bruised clot of many colors.

A BREAKTHROUGH

The fireworks, if any, were positive and occurred in my pre-chemo meeting with Dr. Sitarik. I felt as though I'd experienced a *huge* victory. Up until then, I had been on a strictly palliative track. Dr. Sitarik finally agreed to start me on Avastin, which would target VEGF in tumors. In other words, we were really going to attack these cancers at last, instead of just trying to coddle them into slowing, shrinking, or remaining indolent, if, in fact, they really were indolent.

This new drug came with some significant risk factors—primarily the possibility of fatal bleeds in the brain, lung, and gut. Brain bleeds seem to be related to brain tumors, and I underwent a brain MRI to exclude that possibility. The MRI showed no bleeding in my brain, although it did turn up two probably benign growths in the lining of my brain near the skull. Dr. Sitarik assured me in a series of emails that these growths were fibrous, had sturdy blood vessels, were unlikely to bleed, and therefore were not contraindicated for Avastin.

After doing my research, I discovered that lung bleeds appear to be related to having had lung surgery in the past sixty days, but I was beyond that time frame. Gut bleeds seemed to be attributable to age. As a result of this research, I now had two new definitions of age: "geriatric" is over sixty-five and "elderly" is over seventy. I asked Dr. Sitarik about the error bars on that: "If it's a day before I'm seventy, would you give me the drug?" After much harrumphing around, I think the real answer was that it depended on my individual performance status, a scale that ranges from 0 (yes) to 4 (no way). I was a 1, pretty good for being sixty-nine years old.

I started Avastin the following week and it was to become part of my regular chemo—assuming, of course, that I still would be getting regular chemo. I was scheduled for a CT scan of *everything* on December 10. This, too, was a breakthrough, in my opinion. Before this, no one had looked at anything besides my lungs.

RESEARCH HELP: "TEAM JOANN"

What was the reason for this change in direction? I believe most of it stemmed from the tenacious work of a few good people (as the Marines might say in some future nonsexist era), whom I called "Team Joann." Of note, the hospital librarian provided enthusiastic help, and the volunteers at the Grillo Health Information Center exhibited never-ending patience in researching specific questions.

Another friend, working from Sarasota, joined my research team and found a number of papers that had previously eluded us. Among the most helpful were three or four from a journal called *Expert Opinion*. Following up on both the poster papers and the *Expert Opinion* pieces (opposite ends of the "peer review" spectrum, so to speak), we had garnered some amazing responses.

The librarian at National Jewish Health willingly helped me delve into the mysteries of targeted therapy in a long and trying day there. After I returned to Boulder, she unearthed a paper regarding Alimta maintenance that appeared to at least double survival time for mesothelioma patients, and she forwarded it to me. When I presented Dr. Sitarik with that paper, he read it with interest, noting that some folks were still alive when the paper was written, long after the usual stats say they should be dead. Why was this amazing news not covered in the national media? I think because mesothelioma is so rare. "Only" two thousand patients a year in the United States—that is non-news.

In an attempt to understand the biology involved in targeted therapy, I consulted my friend Abe Flexer, the only biologist I know. Abe, Roger, and I read the abstracts from a late October 2007 conference regarding targeted therapy, identified some likely looking poster papers, and emailed the authors, hoping to find more information on these therapies. "Likely looking" referred to topics such as statins synergistic with taxanes in NSCLC (non-small cell lung carcinoma)—topics that weren't peer reviewed, but might be cutting edge. We used a boiler-plate email that we had worked out: introduction, ask the specific question of the specific researchers, summarize my medical history, sign it with Abe's recognizable name, and hope for the best. The "best" was more than I could have ever hoped for.

Among the replies Abe received was a call from the University of Iowa asking that I call to talk to their researcher. I did, and we agreed that his was probably Plan C. At that point, I was still working on a modification of Plan A, which was to continue my current chemo of Alimta and Carboplatin, and add Avastin to it. But it was comforting to have *options*. Another welcome response was a startlingly nice email from an oncologist at Baylor University in Houston, which concluded: "She is very fortunate to have someone such as you at her side during this difficult time." I agreed and felt very fortunate to have all of my other friends there for me as well.

Then, a reply from a European researcher strongly supported adding a targeted drug. This colleague offered that this drug would soon be the "standard of care." I wondered, *In Europe? Here?* The possible downside was that the drug came in pill form, likely knocking it into the "drug" part of insurance rather than the "Medicare allows" part of insurance. It was unclear how that would shake itself out, but monthly costs for most pill-form targeted therapy ranged from $8,000 to $12,000. Randi Londer Gould's journal, *Community Oncologist*, had quite a bit of helpful information about the Medicare-insurance-drug classification relationship; it was far from a moot point.

RESEARCH FROM FAR AWAY

Dr. Sitarik had been wonderful in his willingness to cooperate with a patient who, with the help of a lot of people, had been trolling the world looking for a better idea. One possible and very encouraging "better idea" was detailed in an email reply to Abe's request from a doctor in Europe. First, Abe's request:

> **Subject:** *Colorado mesothelioma patient*
>
> *Your recent report turned up in my search to help Joann Dennett, a good friend and retired*

colleague from the University of Colorado, Boulder; she is copied on this e-mail. In summer, 2007, Joann was diagnosed with two unrelated cancers: BAC Stage IV (left lung); and mesothelioma (diaphragm and chest wall).

My objective in writing is to ask whether, assuming progressive disease and ineligibility for clinical trials, you might have any suggestions or advice regarding possible treatments or approaches? In particular, might there be a basis for adding bevacizumab to her current therapy (below)? And, if so, whether there is a compelling reason to defer such an addition until she fails current therapy? Also, are there markers that might help resolve this question?

Here are some relevant highlights of her history: Joann, who lives in Boulder, has a history of breast cancer treated aggressively at MDACC by Gabe Hortobagyi in 1980; she has been NED [no evidence of disease] breast cancer since.

As mentioned above, in summer, 2007, Joann was diagnosed with two unrelated cancers: BAC Stage IV (left lung); and mesothelioma— a "large mass" on the diaphragm and "multiple smaller nodules on the chest wall." The former was apparently the "stable nodule in the left lower lobe" that had been followed (PET/CT at MDACC and NJH, Denver) for 14 months. The others were apparently not visible on any of the scans. She is EGFR negative and currently being treated by Mark Sitarik in Boulder with Alitma and Carboplatin. Joann is ineligible for mesothelioma surgery, is 69 years old, in otherwise good health, and performance status 1.

If you have any ideas, suggestions, referrals or insights, Joann and I would certainly be glad to hear them. Please "reply to all."

Thanks in advance for your interest.

I was especially pleased to see that in his email response, the European researcher invited further correspondence and offered a number of ways to achieve that.

I believe that the addition of bevacizumab to the combination of Alimta + Carboplatin is a good idea for two reasons. The first is that Alimta + Carbo/cisplatin in the near future could be a new standard of care in NSCLC especially in adenocarcinoma/BAC histotype and it is now the standard of care for mesothelioma. Chemotherapy + bevacizumab is also a new standard of care for non-squamous NSCLC patients, so it's possible that a three-drug combination Carbo + Alimta + bevacizumab is better than a doublet. The second reason is that we believe that there is a role for bevacizumab in malignant mesothelioma and we are ready to start a clinical trial with this drug. In conclusion, I suggest to try this three-drug combination. No markers are available in clinical practice. At progression I suggest erlotinib independently to the EGFR status.

Feel free to contact me if you have any questions.

Best Regards and Good Luck.

In my opinion, this email was instrumental in moving my treatment forward into targeted therapy territory. The concept of the targeted drug idea seemed to be gaining momentum rapidly. This fueled my main hope that if Avastin targeted therapy for NSCLC could extend survival at this point, perhaps drugs now in the pipeline would come along in time to move NSCLC into the status of chronic and controllable, as the recent advances in colon cancer appear to have done. In other words, I knew Avastin wasn't a cure, but maybe it could keep me around long enough for some real advances to show up. I was really, really glad we were finally going to try it!

When I finally got this treatment, I thought, *I had better be in the 95% it doesn't kill!* And in a small percentage of that 95%, it worked spectacularly. I was ready for spectacular.

NEW IDEAS

By the second week in December 2007, we were back to the drawing board. Unfortunately, the latest CT scan results were not good. At first, Dr. Sitarik said he was waiting for a transcription and that he had asked the transcriptionist to do it *now*. We found out later—much later—that at that point, the radiologist hadn't even looked at my scan yet. While we waited for him to do so, I went off to get my B-12 shot. While getting my shot, I saw the CT tech. She looked at me sadly, maybe with pity. I should have followed up on that look, but I assumed she had seen the report. Wrong assumption. Maybe the pity part was a wrong assumption also.

I got the B-12 shot and then had to use the restroom. Just as I started this private field trip, I remembered that Dr. Sitarik had said he wanted a urine sample to check for excess protein in my urine because of the newly added Avastin. I went down the hall, hunted someone down, and presented my dilemma. She sent me to the lab, but no one was there. Around the corner, I found one of the chemo nurses loading stuff from a closet onto various carts. I told her my predicament and she pointed to someone from the lab standing at the chemo nurse's desk. So I went there, hoping I was not going to wet my pants before I found out how to leave a specimen.

The chemo nurse was talking to a lab person I had not seen before and I re-re-explained my problem. I managed to get a cup and "gathered my sample," but then had the new problem of what to do with it. I wrapped my sample cup in a paper towel and went back to the lab, but still no one was there. So I went back to the room where Roger was sitting. He said no one had been by. I continued on, cup in hand, to find Dr. Sitarik's assistant. She told me to take it back to the lab. I said, "Are they going to take my word for what to do with it?" She said she'd send an order.

Once again I went to the lab, and finally someone was there, but they were helping a person in a wheelchair. I sat down, cup still in hand, to wait. When it was my "turn," I pointed out to the tech who reached for the cup that my name wasn't on it. She scribbled "Dennett, J" on it and I let her have it. *I'm so happy there is a strict protocol to follow for tracking lab samples*, I thought. Then I went back to the room and Roger, who was still reading. It was a good thing that Roger likes to read—he's had a lot of "waiting" time to do that.

Pretty soon, Dr. Sitarik came back to share the initial results of the CT scan from December 10: upper right lung, stable; GGO in left, probably bigger; meso on diaphragm, stable. The written report of the CT scan was contradictory and difficult to understand. The lesions were bigger, but maybe not. After that, Dr. Sitarik said we should stop the chemo. "No point in giving you more cytoxic drugs if they're not working. We'll just give you the Avastin."

I concurred, but I asked, "Aren't they synergistic?"

He thought for a moment and said, "Yes, let's go with two more cycles of chemo." I made a face. He thought some more. We decided to decide later, after he had the full report of the CT scan.

On the way home, I really wasn't happy with that conclusion, and I told Dr. Sitarik so in

The National Comprehensive Cancer Network (NCCN) provides a number of services to physicians. Prominent among them are treatment guidelines for various cancers. They also publish documents called *Up To Date*. These summarize current research and are used by physicians to keep current on topics they may not regularly encounter in their own practices. They can be helpful to the patient as well. To see what topics are available, go to www.uptodate.com.

an email that evening. I started collecting my resources, including the European researcher's paper and email, and a CD with new National Comprehensive Cancer Network (NCCN) guidelines that detail standard treatments for every kind of cancer—every kind of cancer except mesothelioma, that is. It's so frustrating that mesothelioma seems never to get mentioned.

> Ask your physician if *Up To Date* is available to you and request a copy of anything you think you would want to read. If your physician does not have a subscription to *Up To Date*, you can probably obtain copies of topics you would like with a visit to your nearest medical library. Or you can take out a short-term subscription yourself.

Then I started thinking about all of this. It would seem that the synergism of Avastin is with Abraxane and Carboplatin, not Alimta and Carboplatin. *Does this matter?* There's that question again.

The European paper and email suggested Avastin and Tarceva. But did that address *both* cancers? Obviously, I was not in a position to decide. Maybe it was time for the genetic survey surgery.

I was totally full of despair that I was ready for second-line treatment so soon. Second-line treatment starts only when the first treatment regimen fails. To say I was very discouraged is an understatement.

FACING THE REALITY

I decided to try the four-question journaling format from the Seven Levels of Healing workshop again. In mid-December, I pondered the questions with a new, not necessarily better, attitude:

1. How do I feel today? Better because I'm working on a plan. Maybe better because I have no choice. What emotions have I experienced in the last 24 hours? All of them. The CT scan says left BAC is larger. Dread, fear, consternation. Alarm. Tried to talk to Roger about it. He isn't worried. He still thinks I have five good years. Dr. Sitarik did use the word "chronic disease." I'm scared. I think the pain/discomfort in my side is cancer. He thinks it's from the surgery.

2. How do I feel about my cancer? How is it impacting my life? Cancer impacts me always. Today I started this manuscript. Its working title is Ultimate Deadline. I started collating information, and it makes me both nervous and nauseous.

3. What am I willing to give up to heal or to overcome this cancer? I have nothing to give up. I am willing to give up some time. I am willing to commit to exercise to nourish my body. I am willing to work on nutrition again. Are these things I am "giving up"? Seems more to be things I am acquiring.

4. What are the gifts this cancer has brought/can bring to me and my family? Gift?

*Cancer has helped me clear stuff out of my
life. I must soon deal with death issues such
as the church, the hymns I want, Oak Ridge
Cemetery, the obit. Is this a gift—to be done
with it all? If so, a gift for whom?*

My thoughts went back to the night in 1954 when my
father was dying of melanoma at the Army's Walter Reed
Hospital in Washington. Thankfully, my mother did not
fetch me from the couch in the day room. Nonetheless,
from the preceding two months, I knew I did not want to
die the way my father did. I have never coped with his
death, with my helplessness, with his extended suffering,
with his own helplessness. I had hated it when the Army
chaplain came a few days before my father died and read
the Psalm about the Valley of the Shadow of Death. I hid,
hoping they couldn't find me and make me be present. My
father was in an oxygen tent, and the chaplain was there
doing whatever passes for last rites in the Protestant mi-
lieu. The Catholics are lucky, as are the Jews and I suppose
the Muslims. For them, there are rituals—things to do and
say and experience. Protestants seem to just bumble about.
I wondered, *What was my bottom line? Bumbling about?
Total fear?*

*I'll be present at my own death—too soon. I'm not
ready to die. I'm not ready, I'm just not ready.* But the
inevitability of my impending death didn't seem to have
much to do with my readiness. I decided that all I could do

is use the time I had left to create, to leave something behind, to help my husband cope, with both my illness and its aftermath. I felt I had no further necessary responsibilities, only those I was willing to accept.

WHAT IS THE NEXT STEP?

I had been hoping to get my first novel, *See How They Scurry*, out by the end of November 2007, but I settled for a revised goal of early the following year. In December, I was supposed to be doing the cover text for the book, but instead found myself writing down the thoughts that were ever-circling my mind.

How does one face death? We all will. Why was it such a problem for me? Because I wasn't sure if anything I was thinking, saying, or doing was the "right" thing? I wanted to just sit and cry. I thought, *I need a dog to hug and love and cry with.* Unfortunately, for the first time since college, I was dogless.

One week before Christmas, I just felt sad. I was discouraged, unhappy, and had no idea what was going to happen to me. One minute, I was sure it was out of my hands, and the next minute, I decided the reality was that it was up to me to find a treatment that might work.

What I thought I wanted was to wind up on maintenance Alimta, take a full course of Avastin and Tarceva (if

Alimta and Tarceva were compatible with a "vacation from blood issues"), such that I could have the molecular assay Dr. Sitarik had suggested a couple of months prior. I wanted to get the assay done before I turned seventy in September, as that appeared to be some sort of deadline after which I would be "too old."

It was all so complicated, and even more scary was that it was getting harder to think after each chemo. That part worried me. Dr. Sitarik convinced me to stay on chemo. What a Christmas present.

I mused, *How is the cancer impacting my life?* Totally. We haven't been able to enjoy retirement. How do we enjoy what time is left? I didn't want to start new writing projects, but I decided I needed to consider what happens to "things."

Making decisions about "things" actually felt good. Among those things were family furnishings from mid-19th century Illinois—antiques of sentimental if not monetary value. The Iles House in Springfield was happy to get an array of small tables, toys, and rugs that came originally from the home of Sarah Marinda Elliot, my great-great-grandmother, a neighbor of Mary and Abe Lincoln on South 8th Street in Springfield, Illinois.

Then there was a collection of family Bibles, including my maternal grandmother's Smith Family Bible. I managed to find family, albeit distant family, to take these Bibles.

CANCER ISSUES

A few days later, I wondered whether all cancer treatment scenarios were as difficult as mine. It appeared to me that I was dealing with two main issues. First, BAC and mesothelioma do not usually occur together. MD Anderson treats an average of only two cases of mesothelioma a month and "rarely if ever" had seen it coupled with BAC. Dr. Sitarik in Boulder had no prior experience with this challenge. Thank goodness, he readily admitted this and was open to consulting with others and, further, he was open to *me* consulting with others.

Dr. Sitarik was open to *consulting* with others, but he did not seem open to *challenging* his immediate colleagues. I asked that the December CT scan be reread. It didn't happen. Instead, he reread the two scans himself, and discovered that, in at least one instance, the CT report placed a lesion in the right lung (giving coordinates for locating the lesion on the image) that was actually in the left lung (using the image location). I suggested that, given a glaring error *and* the not-quite-right report, we should ask the radiologist to take another look at it. Dr. Sitarik declined.

I then asked him if I could talk to the radiologist directly. He said no. I should not have asked him first and wouldn't make that error in the future. But, once he said no, I didn't see how I could ignore his order and call the radiologist anyway.

I was feeling the effects of the chemo more and more. One could argue that such misery would be worth it were there a light at the end of the tunnel. In my case, there *was* a light, but I was convinced it was an oncoming train. I debated the wisdom of continuing chemo. Dr. Sitarik reminded me that I chose to attempt treatment when he offered to wait for symptoms.

Given the lack of clarity of the report from the last CT scan, I decided to appeal to the good will of Dr. Buether and ask National Jewish for a second opinion.

> *Hi:*
>
> *Would it be possible for your radiologist to look at my last two CT scans done up here in Boulder and tell me what he thinks?*
>
> *I have CDs of these scans. They were done 10/30 and 12/10. The report of the 10/30 says, in part, that the lesions in the right lung are smaller and everything else is stable. It also compares this scan with those done at NJH in Jan and June.*
>
> *The report of 12/10 is pretty jumbled in the text . . . it actually reads as though the radiologist at BCH was interrupted in his dictation and forgot where he was when he resumed . . . the summary says "probably larger" GGO but rest stable. (But that's not what the*

jumbled text appears to say . . . it mentions growth in several places. Further, it does not compare this scan to the NJH scans but only to the one six weeks prior.)

Anyway, since these two scans are being used as the basis for deciding whether to maintain me on Alimta/Carboplatin for two more cycles (five and six) or to switch drugs, I'd be a whole lot more comfortable with a second opinion.

Thank you for your thoughts and, I hope, help.

Joann

As usual with Dr. Buether, I quickly received a reply:

Joann,

One of my nurses will call you next week, probably Mon or Wed.

To do this, we will need you to mail us the 2 CT scans to my attention. Then, I'd like to see you in clinic at least 1 week after we get the CT scan, because it takes that long for an official radiology interp.

If this timeline doesn't work for your decision making, let the nurses know that when they call—I don't want to waste your time. My schedule is also a mess, because I am out mid-Jan for 2 weeks, so we may have to bail on the clinic visit if we can't squeeze you in, and just send you the radiology interp.

Have a happy holiday season!

Dave

LAST CHEMO
(FOR THE TIME BEING)

January 10, 2008, was my last day of chemo. *Great! I'm done!* Except that it was starting to seem as if the chemo hadn't really worked, and we were back to the "watch and wait" game. I envied my email friend who'd had such great success with chemo that he was getting treatments currently being denied to me: Cyberknife, Tarceva, and who knows what else. In my case, each round of chemo was harder than the last, seemed to cause more new problems, and made me crabbier than the one before. This time, bleeding (a dog bumps me, and I bleed) and peripheral neuropathy moving over from the central nervous system to the major motor nerves (the ones that help you do things like stand and walk) seemed to be the latest and greatest of the new symptoms.

The problem with worsening motor skills manifested itself big-time not long thereafter when I simply could not get out of a chair at a friend's home. My quads just sat there and said, "No way. Forget it." Then, the next day, I couldn't get out of the car. Next, I stumbled in the living room and nearly fell. It was really beginning to scare me, and all I could think of was, *If I can't get out of a chair, how would I ever get off the floor?*

So I began using a walker, stopped going out in the snow, put new energy into doing the exercises the physical therapist gave me in order to engage the motor muscles, and generally became even more annoyed. My physical therapist felt the need to comment. "Well, you are heavy, you know. It's hard work for your quads to stand up." I felt the need to point out that I had a pretty fat butt for forty years or so and have never had trouble standing up or walking before. *Grrr.*

Over the last ten years or so, I've had occasional issues with racing heart (tachycardia). I initially described it as "a square wave function." In other words, one beat it's normal (79 for me) and the next, it's 130. This occurred very occasionally, maybe once or twice a year, and lasted for a few hours.

Then, early in 2008, it happened and didn't quit. I finally went to the ER, they did a CT scan and found lots of pulmonary emboli. So I wound up in the intensive care unit (ICU) for a few days. The treatment was blood-thinning shots. And an admonition against flying for 90 days.

STILL LOOKING FOR ALTERNATIVES

The European doctor continued his correspondence with Abe and looked at parts of my last two CT scans. He thought I was getting "excellent results," hoped "patient stays on treatment," and was still recommending six to eight rounds of Carboplatin along with Alimta and Avastin if "patient can tolerate it." (The patient did *not* think she could tolerate it.)

I also sent my last three CT scans to Dr. Buether at National Jewish. He and his "best radiologist in the world" both thought that the chemo *was* working and that I should continue with it.

I wondered what Dr. Sitarik would have to say after seeing the next CT scan. My opinion was that, unless this chemo had made significant progress in reducing my tumor load, we would have to find a different solution. (I defined "significant" as gone or almost gone—not 25% reduction, as the radiologist defined it.) Interestingly, the National Jewish radiologist actually measured the "significantly" reduced lesion to four significant figures. Given that the lesion in question was a GGO, a starburst of light that doesn't have regular margins, I could not imagine how he measured four significant figures nor, therefore, what his measurements actually meant.

At that point, I didn't even know *what* to hope for except to be able to walk safely again.

CHAPTER FIVE

ATTACKING THE MESOTHELIOMA

By mid-March 2008, I still had pain, plus now I had a lump in my side. At about this time, I came across an article about radiofrequency ablation (RFA) and found a glimmer of hope. *Who does it?* I wondered. *Maybe Mayo? Why not for me? Too many lesions. Maybe not BAC? What? Why?* It seemed to me that there was so much to be discovered and too much indolence on the part of anyone but me in trying to discover it.

The day before my appointment with Dr. Sitarik on March 25, I was so nervous that it was hard to sleep. I worried about the discomfort, the lump, the new pain in my left side. But Dr. Sitarik said simply, "No change, come back in three months." *Whew.* But I didn't feel like whew. Besides, I was *really* in pain where Dr. Sitarik dug hard into my side.

Wait and see. I knew the meso was with me. I had pain in my shoulder, pain in my left side, aching pain on lying down. Some nights, gas pains were so extreme that I slept in a chair. But I knew I needed to enjoy these three chemo-free months, so I filled my calendar with things I liked to do.

In early April 2008, I saw *La Boheme* with a couple of good friends. How great to be able to sit and enjoy it, but Mimi's impending death was an uncomfortable few minutes for me. *A little too close to home.*

PLANNING A CHANGE OF VENUE

Roger and I decided a change of venue was in order. We were hoping to go to Connecticut to the graduation of a good friend's daughter in June, and since it seemed a reasonable expectation, we decided to make it the final stop of a month-long journey to Europe. I wasn't supposed to fly because of the possibility of blood clots, so instead we decided we would take the train from Denver to Chicago and then on to New York.

Part two of this planned vacation would take us to Southhampton, England, on the Queen Mary II. Ten days in England, then the train would take us under the English Channel to Paris where we would take a river cruise up the Seine from Paris to Honfleur—simply glorious. I could hardly wait.

After Paris, I would be cleared to fly, and so we would return stateside for the graduation in Connecticut. What a wonderful and much-needed reprieve full of friends, family, and fun. Finally, we would return home just in time for my next CT scan in June.

"Wait and see" felt very much like the previous two years when MD Anderson and National Jewish were doing scans every three months. If either cancer started to grow again, it would be time for Plan B, whatever that might be. At that moment, Plan B consisted solely of working on finding an option that wouldn't destroy my quality of life (QOL) again. If the CT scan after our vacation in June still showed stable disease, then I would have another three months without worry, that time with the goal of attending my "baby" cousin's wedding in Springfield, Illinois, in October.

AN UNEXPECTED ADDITION
TO OUR TRIP PLANS

An Employee Health Survey was being conducted through the union at NASA Lewis (now Glenn) Research Center, where I had worked in the sixties. A suspected cancer cluster had been determined and, in May 2008, I was in contact with a law firm in Los Angeles who represented mesothelioma victims.

They suggested that I consult with a physician at UCLA who performed a different sort of surgery for mesothelioma. I talked to someone at the surgeon's facility at length, and he determined that because I had two primary cancers, I wasn't a candidate for this surgery. I went back to trying to figure out what to pack for my much anticipated five-week journey. Then someone from the law firm called and suggested that I talk to the nurse practitioner at the Mesothelioma Applied Research Foundation (MARF). I called MARF, left a message, and went back to packing. She quickly called back, saying I absolutely needed to see Dr. Robert Taub at Columbia-Presbyterian Medical Center in New York. She gave me the number, and said she would call ahead to say I would be calling. So, after putting the wash in the dryer, I called and got Dr. Taub's assistant. Could she call me right back? *Yeah, right.* But call back she did and quickly. Red flags were starting to wave in the back of my mind. *What is going on here?*

I explained to Dr. Taub's assistant that I was going to Europe shortly, that I would be in Connecticut on June 4 and 5, had pretty much given up on anyone doing anything about the mesothelioma, and that I was not excited about coming back to New York once I got home from vacation. Her response, "Fine, Dr. Taub will see you at 4:00 p.m. on June 5." Then she sent me an eight-page list of information they wanted from me, all at various times: some in the next two weeks, some in the week before I was to arrive and some to bring with me. *Not happening,* I thought. I immediately emailed back and said, "I can't do this. You'll have to get it all at once and keep track of it. I'm not hauling extra stuff around Europe, and I might lose it anyway." So it went all together by FedEx. I went back to packing.

HEADING EAST

We left Denver by train on a pleasant warm evening. The home team Rockies were playing. Our sleeper cabin was far from the station, almost up to the ball field. We got a shuttle ride from the railroad station to our sleeper car, waved goodbye to the friends who drove us to the station from Boulder, and watched them drive off in our van.

On board, we rushed to dinner because the dining car was closing soon. Nice salmon meal. We talked with a couple from Estes Park. They ride Amtrak everywhere and buy everything possible with their Amtrak credit card in order to get points for free Amtrak travel.

Back in our cabin, the beds were made. Getting into the cabin was tricky because the unfolded beds filled up the doorway. But once in, the cabin wasn't too crowded. The bathroom, however, reminded me of Star Trek's teletransporter, or maybe a round coffin—I prefer the teletransporter analogy.

Poor Rog had trouble getting into the top bunk. There was no head room and it's really hard for him to bend his artificial knee, so he wound up sort of flinging himself onto the bed. There were straps to attach to the ceiling so he couldn't fall out.

We met a couple from Wellington, New Zealand, the next morning at breakfast. They were visiting what they called the "Big Four." On inquiry, they said this was New York, San Francisco, Las Vegas, and Chicago. Maybe it was Los Angeles, not San Francisco—I was so amazed by the inclusion of Las Vegas I think I stopped listening.

When we arrived in Chicago, I had my first experience handling my own luggage. Pink carry-on secured on top of rolling suitcase in left hand, fanny pack around waist, coat tied around neck, cane in right hand. It worked!

I was mobile and reasonably speedy until we got into the station. Union Station has many commuter lines. People were running in all possible directions. Hundreds of people who knew where they were going and I, who had no idea where I was going. I cowered against a wall, trying to read the signs (which, of course, was difficult because I couldn't see very well anymore). Rog pulled up behind me and said, "Keep moving." Where?

Just then, a lady stopped and said, "Weren't you on a sleeper?" I said, "Yes," and she said, "Follow me." We did just that and wound up at the First Class Lounge. There you can leave your luggage, sit down, re-find your bearings, and check in for the next train. We did all this and then we boarded the next train one and a half hours before it left. In the First Class Lounge at 7:30 p.m. or so, they had announced something to the effect of "We won't be boarding very early," and then about 10 minutes later, they announced boarding. Again, we got a shuttle ride to our sleeper car. They had wine, cheese, and grapes set up in the dining car. We had to ask the conductor to put the beds down. We were tucked in well before we left Chicago. This time, the upper bunk was easier for Rog. He had three to four feet of space above the bunk *and* a handhold on the wall. He could turn and sit down on the bed. He also had his own window up there. Much better.

I started to experience severe intestinal distress after leaving Chicago, and I felt only mildly better upon arriving in Penn Station. About 10:00 that evening, it became clear that I was really ill. I called Rocky Mountain Cancer Center in Boulder and was told I could take as many as eight Imodium pills a day, but if I was not better in the morning, I needed to seek local medical advice.

I was sick all night with copious vomiting, diarrhea, shaking chills, and high fever. All hallmarks of gallbladder problems, although no one recognized it at that time. It was easy to write the symptoms off to my body recovering from large amounts of chemo.

The next morning, I was able to speak with the hotel's "on-call" doctor. We discussed the likelihood that I was dehydrated. He said I could come to his office for a shot to stop the vomiting, but I would need to go to the emergency room first for intravenous fluids. He offered to call ahead to tell them I was on my way. I then called the office of Dr. Taub, the meso specialist I was to see June 5 at Columbia-Presbyterian, and spoke to his assistant. Her answer to my problem: "Get in a taxi and go to the emergency room at Roosevelt Hospital right now."

And so we went. Assuming I had a virus, the ER isolated me, gave me IV fluids, did blood work, took a urine sample, and then wanted a stool sample. I couldn't "produce" a stool sample for them the way I had multiple times before arriving in the ER. It didn't help either that I had to trek through the ER three, four, five times holding the IV bag and trying to keep my gown shut to get to the ladies' room. Eventually they let me go, and I returned to the hotel with a prescription for nausea and the remnants of a fever.

That night, the diarrhea finally stopped after the maximum eight Imodium for the day, but then the fever, chills, and shaking started up again. *What to do?* We were to embark on the Queen Mary II the next day. I started worrying about the trip and whether we should cancel. I *hated* the idea. But this wasn't just my usual stress before travel, and this was a huge, complicated trip with many places to go. I was worried.

Sadly, by the next day, it was clear the Queen Mary II would sail without us. My fever was down to 100 and I had only occasional chills, but the diarrhea was back with a vengeance. I made the call to the cruise line to cancel, hoping we'd be able to reschedule soon.

Back to my larger issues: If I have a severely limited time to live, I am not happy about wasting time doing things I don't want to do. What I wanted to do was go home. But I felt I *must* see Dr. Taub at Columbia-Presbyterian first. After all, I *was* already on the East Coast. I was recovering enough for us to stay there, so we headed to Connecticut for an early, unexpected visit.

After four days, with me clearly on the mend, we set out for an unplanned driving "tour." Our first stop was Gettysburg. At Gettysburg, honor and God are big, as I guess is true at all war sites. The museum was well done. There were many places to sit down and watch "films" and hear more about honor. For example, the Governor of Pennsylvania had called for all men in Pennsylvania to honor the 35,000 who have died in defense of Pennsylvania—and meet Lee's invading army so thousands more could die. The deaths on both sides were horrifically huge.

We stopped at the Resource Center and played with the data bases there. One of them, "The Faces of Gettysburg," lets you click on one of the "faces" and see what happened to the individuals pictured. I explored a few. The officers (captains, majors, lieutenants) were "mortally wounded" but lived 10 to 40 days before ultimately dying of their wounds. Enlisted men seemed to die instantly or, at the most, overnight. This was *not* a comprehensive survey, just my random observation. *But* it did raise a few questions. Were enlisted men wounded more? And helped less? Roger said it was because officers were on horses behind the front lines and perhaps not as badly wounded.

After Gettysburg, we roamed around until we wound up in Maine. Roger had always said his family's roots were in Maine. However, it was a shock to discover just how widespread those roots were. The first Maine exit on I-95 is Dennett Road. The phone books have columns of Dennetts, and I took a picture of Roger standing in front of a street sign that marked the intersection of Old Dennett Road and New Dennett Road.

Later, in Bath, a visit to the local genealogical society produced much information about Roger's immediate family. We found the site of his great-grandfather's store and the cemetery markers for his great-grandparents in town and his great-great-grandparents on Starbird Road, well out of town, almost to Bowdoin.

On Memorial Day 2008, we had arrived at the Precision Tool Museum in Windsor, Vermont. There I learned that the first modern assembly line was one for producing rifles. It was interesting, certainly quiet and peaceful. It gave me time to think about Memorial Day, and again about my father and his horrific death from cancer in 1954.

MEETING DR. TAUB

What was my hope in seeing Dr. Taub? Some kind of new assessment of my status. Maybe even some idea of what to do and where to do it. I questioned my motives. *What do I want?* I wanted not to be sick. Apparently, that was not possible. Failing that, I wanted a long-term plan, a really *long* long-term plan. Five to ten years seemed like a lifetime at that point. I wanted to be able to travel—maybe even take the Queen Mary II at the last minute sometime.

Finally June 5 arrived and Roger and I met with Dr. Taub. After our initial consultation, I was encouraged, but

Roger wasn't. I had heard Dr. Taub say there was something that could be done, but I had also heard all of the things he would *not* do for me. Roger had heard only "palliative." Palliative didn't just mean living pain free; it might really just mean only a delay of the inevitable.

Dr. Taub had also said the BAC *could* be a long time growing. He spent some time looking at scans before he raised the issue of pleural thickening. I mentioned two bouts of pleurisy I had experienced decades ago. He suggested looking at older scans to see whether the thickening had appeared on those.

TRYING TO KEEP GOING

The following day was graduation day for our friend's daughter in Connecticut. This was the precipitating reason we had come to the East Coast. I looked in the mirror while brushing my teeth and, for the first time, saw death looking back at me.

On a positive note, graduation day was also the day my first novel, *See How They Scurry*, was published. It had been a learning process for me and all the friends who helped me through my first venture in self-publishing.

When we returned to Boulder that weekend, I was still unwell. I was frustrated, and I was tired of being sick and tired. This feeling of unwellness had been going on for months now and, as it turns out, was incorrectly attributed to my cancers. It wasn't long before fever and chills landed me in the hospital. In an effort to seek some comfort from others who could understand, I reached out to my friends:

> *The last six-plus weeks have been difficult, not because of the cancer but because of an on-going saga of issues/extreme fevers/dehydration/chills and shakes that neared the level of seizure a few times. It was one of the latter that sent me to the ER for the second time in 18 hours last Saturday afternoon. I have been in the hospital from then until yesterday. After every possible scan, culture, and myriad blood tests, the diagnosis is FUO (fever of unknown origin).*
>
> *It probably started in New York when we had to cancel out on the Queen Mary. I eventually subdued it there, sort of, but it apparently incubated for four weeks and then just exploded. Hopefully it will not survive four days of IV Merrem (new, ultra-potent antibiotic) and the current ten days of Keflex.*
>
> *Joann*

QUESTIONING THE CURRENT PLAN

I looked back to my current doctors and existing treatment plan. I liked Dr. Sitarik. Rocky Mountain Cancer Center seemed to be taking very good care of me, but I thought they were totally focused on one pervasive mindset: She will die. Let's do no further harm until we have to treat overt symptoms.

Meanwhile, I continued my research in the medical literature. I read in more detail about possible treatments (frying tumors, tomotherapy, Alimta maintenance). I heard from my email friend who had opted for both Cyberknife surgery and EGFR. He had been holding his own with no apparent return of either cancer until July. Then both cancers not only returned, but they were as big as they had been in the beginning. He died a few weeks later.

At various points, Dr. Sitarik had said:

1. I could reasonably expect to live one year.

2. My cancer(s) were slow growing and may not grow for months or even years.

3. If they continued to grow, if the disease continued to worsen . . .

As I understood his current plan, we would wait for the inevitable growth and then get tissue for a molecular assay. One paper I found talked of a collection of six different people who had meso and who had had their tumors assayed. The results had little in common with each other, so assay of my meso would surely be a good idea. Otherwise, it seemed that treatment could be little better than throwing a dart at a moving target.

Waiting for the BAC to grow did *not* seem like such a good idea. Radiofrequency ablation seemed like a better idea. Why wait for new lesions to manifest? RFA was repeatable and almost outpatient. But Dr. Sitarik had said no because the procedure is particularly hard on the host—that is, on me.

MY GALLBLADDER

The doctors in Boulder finally figured out what had been making me so sick for so long. Gallstones, not cancers, were the root of my problem. Surgery on July 21, 2008, successfully removed my gallbladder, but a continual IV drip during and after surgery filled my body with excess fluid. My heart couldn't deal with that much excess fluid and quit working very well. My B-type natriuretic peptide (BNP) blood test, which measures the risk for congestive heart failure, peaked above 1800 (a normal reading is 125) before someone prescribed something to help eliminate the extra fluid and bring relief to my struggling heart. As of the next morning, I had managed to pee away seventeen and a half pounds of weight in fluid alone.

A visit to Rocky Mountain Cancer Center left my care team scratching their heads. No one could believe I had gained and lost so much so fast. The physician's assistant wanted to know, "Does your scale work?" My BNP was blessedly back down to 127. The computer at the doctor's office flagged this 127 test result as "high." Ha! It should see HIGH!

I was exhausted and depressed—big-time depressed. I had planned to take the week off to recuperate and read. Mostly, I slept and stared into space. I still wanted to go to Europe. Did I want to go to Illinois to visit family? That seemed less important now than staying in Boulder, where my friends were providing the support I needed.

The next month, a bout with tachycardia while visiting the cardiologist landed me in the ICU for several days. At one point, I looked over to see Roger trying to sleep in the chair in my room. He was propped on one fist with a scowl of pain on his face. Pain, exhaustion, sorrow. What is this doing to us? To both of us, not just me.

BAD NEWS/GOOD NEWS

By September 2008, much had changed. The BAC in my left lung had grown by 10% since June. Dr. Sitarik sent my pathology slides and blocks to Target Now in Phoenix, which tries to ascertain which drugs to prescribe for an individual's specific tumor.

Where there is bad news, however, sometimes there comes good news. What was assumed to be BAC in my right lung, either mets or a second primary, had disappeared. A cascade of logic as to why it was gone materialized: if it disappeared, it wasn't cancer; if it wasn't cancer, I never had Stage IV BAC in my right lung; if I didn't have Stage IV BAC, then I was a candidate for curative surgery.

A CHANCE TO CHOOSE

I didn't have Stage IV lung cancer in my right lung. I couldn't believe it. Ecstatic didn't even begin describe how I felt. For just a moment, I managed to forget that the BAC in my left lung was still growing. But, since it was never there in the right lung, the left lung was still operable (resectable, as the medical folks say), and maybe the lung cancer was not terminal.

I felt as though I had been handed my life back. I was given the chance to choose the best thing to do with it. All options were back on the table. Obviously, the first "option" was to get rid of the lung cancer. Operable Stage IB BAC has a survival rate of 50% at five years. *Way* different from the 2% for Stage IV, but not as good as it might have been when it was Stage IA last year.

Don't look back, I thought.

But I still had mesothelioma. So it was still possible that doctors would not operate to remove the BAC in my left lung "in the face of the mesothelioma," as Dr. Sitarik said. However, Dr. Taub at Columbia-Presbyterian, who had just started a new clinical trial of what he called "The Columbia Protocol vs. mesothelioma," agreed that I was a candidate for his protocol, but not the clinical trial.

COLUMBIA-PRESBYTERIAN DECISION

Roger and I flew to New York to reconfer with the Columbia-Presbyterian team. Even though I liked the surgeon at Columbia-Presbyterian and Dr. Taub and everyone on his team, I did not like New York. Not even a little. Manhattan is difficult for someone with my limited mobility, and we spent a lot of money on transportation. This would be the downside of treatment there. Getting around, finding a place to stay, and eating out all the time might be more than we were prepared to take on.

But the benefits outweighed everything else, and we agreed to treatment at Columbia-Presbyterian. The surgery sounded horrific, but it offered the only hope of a significantly extended life. I had a long conversation with Dr. Taub regarding my concerns about treatment and surgery, and although he remained patient with me, I was frustrated by his increasing insistence on asking me to "trust" him. I wasn't sure that the copious questions I was asking were the same as mistrust, and I pondered how trust had become an issue. *Not the same issue here*, I thought. I hoped not.

PREPARATION FOR SURGERY

The Crowne Plaza Hotel in Englewood, New Jersey, offered special rates for Columbia-Presbyterian patients. We arrived there in October 2008 for a week of preliminary testing before surgery. It was less than ideal, requiring an involved shuttle ride to the hospital. We contemplated other accommodations and the possibilities for the longer upcoming stay after surgery. If everyone involved agreed to move forward with surgery and subsequent treatment, it was possible we would be in New York as long as sixteen weeks.

The hospital also had rooms available for family. These were expensive but would put Roger only an elevator ride away from my hospital bed. So it could be a solution for a few days. But after that, where would we stay? Probably we would move around trying a bit of this and a bit of that. For now, though, we settled down in New Jersey.

The hotel shuttle between New Jersey and Columbia-Presbyterian ran on a limited schedule with only three options: 9:00 a.m., 11:30 a.m., and 8:00 p.m. This meant we had to ride in on the first van in order to keep my 11:00 a.m. appointment with the Columbia surgeon. When the alarm went off at 7:00 that first morning, my body insisted it was barely 5:00 in the morning, which, of course, it was in Colorado.

On the shuttle that morning, we met a young couple who had been in New York for six months. He was being treated for meso by Dr. Taub, and it was encouraging that they could not say enough wonderful things about the treatment and the Columbia doctors. This couple also offered a lot of advice about housing, ending with the observation that the Crowne Plaza was indeed the best deal.

Upon quizzing them, I found that their "best deal" judgment was based largely on the free breakfast and nightly hors d'oeuvres offered to high-level Priority Club members.

Our forced early arrival at the hospital coupled with a long wait in an overly hot waiting room produced two very sleepy people for our first meeting with the surgeon. If he agreed to operate on the BAC in my left lung, Dr. Taub would work with him on the meso at the same time, making for a very long surgery. This could be a problem for both Roger and me. A problem for me because I'd had a lot of surgery recently. A problem for Roger because he would have to sit, wait, and worry in a place where he knew no one.

I also thought I had an appointment with Dr. Taub that afternoon, but on arriving I found that he was in synagogue all day for the High Holidays. An appointment was made for the next day. Next was the task of figuring out how to get "home" back across the George Washington Bridge. The hotel van would have been only $24 but it wasn't coming for seven more hours. We opted for a twelve-minute cab ride at a cost of nearly $100. We both went right to bed. I slept for several hours; Roger took his usual forty-minute midday nap.

Remembering the advice from the couple on the morning shuttle about the fantastic hors d'oeuvres awaiting us in the hotel penthouse, we reported there promptly at

6:00 p.m. and filled up on coconut shrimp, fresh fruit, and cheese. They were right—it was delicious, filling, and free.

A LOT OF UNKNOWNS

A lot of unknowns still lurked, any one of which could derail my current treatment plan: my multiple comorbidities for surgery (notably my heart, high body mass index, and previous pulmonary emboli), plus the fact that within one week I would be over seventy and into the medically defined realm of "elderly." Also, the meso could be more advanced than anyone expected. (At that time, Dr. Taub used his protocol only on "early" meso.) Those were the potential problems that I knew about; probably there were many others about which I knew nothing.

But still I was encouraged because Dr. Taub's protocol had been effective against peritoneal meso. His published paper of February 20, 2008 (M. Hesdorffer, first author), showed a median survival of more than sixty months. It was a small testing sample (thirty people or so), and nine people had died quickly. The sixty-month median was even more impressive, since it included the nine near-immediate deaths.

MORE GOOD NEWS

The week we spent at Columbia-Presbyterian was a busy one and, pending the results of a complete pulmonary function test done at the altitude where I want to live—that is, in Boulder, more than a mile above sea level—I was finally deemed to be a candidate for surgery.

As I would not be part of any clinical trial, the surgeon had said they would do "whatever is best for you" once they got the lung cancer out, which would involve the partial removal of my left lung (lobectomy). Then Dr. Taub's treatment would start with intrapleural chemo, a direct application of hot chemo into the pleural space around my lungs, before I left the operating room.

For that whole week we spent in New York, I had been getting increasingly nervous about the plan for surgery and treatment there. *Why*? I was pretty sure it was mostly about the hassle of being in Manhattan, getting around Manhattan in less than ideal shape, keeping Roger from going nuts, and keeping me from the same.

Yet, when I thought about it rationally, it seemed to be my only hope for, *dare I say*, beating the meso. Probably not a reasonable hope, but, there it was. I hoped that Columbia-Presbyterian's treatment would knock the meso back for enough years that something curative would come along. With this in mind, I didn't want to slam any doors to possible future treatment. We returned to Colorado and waited for a surgery date.

SURGERY

A month later, with a surgery date in place, we left for New York with trepidation as well as high hopes. My surgery on October 23, 2008, went well. The surgeon removed the left lower lobe of my lung and put catheters in my chest for Dr. Taub to pour chemo directly onto the mesothelioma lesions on my chest wall. But, before that, the first use of the catheters was to circulate a heated chemo drug (cisplatin) into and out of my thoracic space for an hour. Mercifully I was out cold in the operating room while this was going on.

The operation went smoothly; recovery, however, was a nightmare. The hospital was understaffed, overloaded, whatever you want to call it. It was truly frightening to be in the ICU for two days, unable to move and totally dependent on apparently overworked and crabby people. Further, my room was next to a door that people went through frequently, and each time, the door slammed loudly.

I was approved for food after a day, but none ever came. Who knew why not? It had been ordered, but when it didn't come, no one did anything. Finally, one of the staff took pity on me and got me a box of food from the deli in the hospital lobby at its closing time. It was a measure of my desperation that, at 11:00 that night, I ate a stale egg salad sandwich.

During this time, Roger was trying to "commute" between our hotel across the George Washington Bridge in

New Jersey and the hospital. Since the last shuttle left the hospital at 8:15 p.m., visiting hours, which started at 8:00, weren't very useful. My last night in the ICU, Roger was in my room at 7:00, when someone decided to revel in their "power over all" and came to tell Roger that it was illegal for him to be there because they were going to do rounds and he might overhear something about another patient. *Bull-crackers.* Groups of people had frequently stopped outside my door and discussed me and my case in loud voices. Who had "overheard" those discussions? Anyone and everyone within earshot.

Threatened with a call to security, Roger left my bedside and I started my last night alone in the ICU. My last lucid observation was when my next door neighbor died and the cart from the morgue came to get her. I hit my pain button—not because I hurt, but because I didn't want to be where I was anymore. An IV jolt of Dilaudid guaranteed unconsciousness.

When I actually was moved out of the ICU the following day, it was to a step-down unit with four beds and, supposedly, better monitoring. I did have more monitors on, if that is how "better monitoring" is measured. My immediate neighbor, three feet from my bed behind a curtain, screamed almost constantly. The poor woman, as far as I could tell, got little attention from anyone other than her family. The beds across the room were occupied by men. The guy across from me got a great deal of attention. He got to brush his teeth in the morning, had his hair combed, sat up, and got a food tray. My vitals were taken every six or eight hours, I continued to get only leftover food that Rog shared, and that was it. I decided the guy across the way must have a private-pay nursing assistant, but Roger countered that there was no private-pay care allowed in step-down units. In retrospect, it was interesting that the surgeon had actually suggested we consider hiring a private-duty nurse. The hospital itself even has an office to help you do this. That should have been a clue to the level of care on the floor.

On the last day, I was transferred into a regular room. It was fairly pleasant and I got a food tray, a menu, and a bath. It had been four days since my surgery. The next morning, when the doctor asked me if I wanted to go home, I said "Yes," even though at that point "home" was a hotel.

Back at the hotel, we hired a private-duty nurse to stay with me the first night in an adjoining room. Roger got a room all to himself on a different floor, and got a good night's sleep for the first time since my surgery. The nurse cost us $800 for the night, but it was better than being in that nightmare hospital one more night.

HOPE LODGE

While I was "recovering" in the hotel, we learned that we had been accepted into the American Cancer Society's Hope Lodge. We moved into Hope Lodge as soon as we could, and it was wonderful. We had a lovely room, reminiscent of the quality of a high-end hotel: two twin beds, a sitting area with couch and chair, a TV that unfortunately could be viewed well only from the toilet, and a large wheelchair-accessible bathroom.

Hope Lodge is located in the American Cancer Society (ACS) building on 32nd Street West. It turned out to be a great place to interact with other patients, exchange information, and gain support. The constant concern, caring, and support offered by staff and other patients and families was truly wonderful. The best part of Hope Lodge? It was free, thanks to the ACS.

Hope Lodges are owned and operated by the American Cancer Society in various major cities. They provide free housing for out-of-town cancer patients undergoing long-term treatment. Similar free or low-cost housing options are detailed on www.joeshouse.org, a nonprofit lodging guide that offers a nationwide list of places for out-of-town cancer patients to stay while being treated.

To explore other options in specific cities, check online or with a social worker where you are being treated.

Aside from having comfortable rooms, we had access to a laundry room and a large community area with a computer center, meditation room, a TV with Wii games, and a library. Not quite home, but certainly better than the hotel. There was also a huge community kitchen on each floor with two sets of stoves, a refrigerator, microwave, spices, dishes, utensils, and an eating area. We were responsible for buying and making our own food, and the challenge quickly became finding a place to shop. The first time Roger went out, he came back with just a jar of instant coffee. Online, we located a Whole Foods Market, but it was six good-sized blocks away—a very long way to carry groceries.

After some time at Hope Lodge, we developed a system with other patients and their families for meal making, taking turns making large meals for lots of people. Even Roger took his turn, making his "famous" cheese chicken.

The distance between Hope Lodge and the hospital was a problem, however, especially as I got sicker with the on-going weekly chemo. When I had chemo appointments at Columbia-Presbyterian, it was necessary to take a car service. This cost about $50 each way. Further, they allowed us to set up a charge account, which meant we didn't have to carry much cash, a good thing in New York.

And it was certainly necessary. As each weekly treatment made me more ill, knowing we were almost an hour from the Columbia-Presbyterian ER became more and more unsettling. Also, the fact that Roger could not stay at Hope Lodge without me if I wound up in the hospital again was scary. These thoughts consumed a lot of what little energy I had left.

UNBEARABLE CHEMO

I had such pain after the chemo was poured into the catheters in my chest that I cried and tried not to scream all the way back to Hope Lodge after each treatment. Alas, after the third treatment, I decided that I couldn't bear any more. This was only halfway through the planned chemo, and Dr. Taub and I exchanged lengthy emails about my decision to quit. Nonetheless, my final decision was not to continue with this unbearable chemo any longer, and we went home to Boulder.

We arrived in Boulder on December 10, 2008, almost too late. I was seriously ill. This became undeniably apparent on the flight home. I was taking Dilaudid, Tylenol, and Vicodin to make the trip possible. And I went to bed for more than a week once we got home. I roused for a trip to the local surgeon to get the catheters in my chest removed, and I was able to rouse myself once again for Christmas.

Loved ones tried to share their holiday joy with us. Friends joined us on Christmas Eve, bringing dinner and gifts. Still others came on Christmas Day, also with dinner and gifts.

On Boxing Day, I finally gave up and went to Rocky Mountain Cancer Center. That afternoon, I was admitted to BCH, having been diagnosed with two empyemas, painful buildups of infection in my chest.

New Year's Day 2009 found me still in the hospital, where I would remain for another eleven days before being released. Once home, I needed a daily IV antibiotic for

> For expenses that are not covered by Medicare, and for which you are billed the entire (and probably overwhelming) amount, contact the billing department of the provider to negotiate a lower cost. Start by offering *immediate payment* of whatever Medicare would have paid had it been covered. (You don't have to know what that is; they will know.) Your offer to pay immediately is important. Do it even if you have to finance the cost.

several more weeks. Roger was trained in how to administer this antibiotic through the existing PICC (peripherally inserted central catheter) line in my arm. Once a week, Walgreens delivered the drug and supplies to the front door.

All was well until we got the pharmacy bill. It was more than $19,000 for the drug. Medicare didn't cover it because it was administered at home and not in a medical setting. Since Medicare didn't cover it, my Medigap also didn't. We were stuck with the whole bill. That is, we were stuck until a friend who works at a local Hospice made a suggestion.

Taking her suggestion, I called the Walgreens number in Illinois, from whence the dunning phone calls were coming, and made them an offer. "I will pay whatever Medicare would have paid, had they paid. And I will pay it today if you will accept that." They did. The bill was a little over $2,000. Still a lot, but not as much as $19,000.

Barak Obama was inaugurated on January 20, 2009. I sat in a chair and watched the whole thing on TV. The oath and festivities at the Capitol, the drive, the parade. And perhaps because I was sitting for so long I got a blood clot at the outlet of the PICC line. So more hassle of back and forth to the hospital. Finally, they pulled the PICC line out and decreed that I had received enough antibiotic. And I was done with that.

The next step was radiation to deter the lesion of mesothelioma on the nerve that controls my diaphragm function. That too was a lesson in Medicare payments. The surgeon at Columbia-Presbyterian had wisely put in gold beads to mark the location of this lesion for future targeting of radiation. The decision was to use Cyber-knife, which is not a knife at all but very focused radiation. The radiation beam is directed at the target lesion from more than 100 different angles, thus assuring that the healthy tissue around the lesion is not overradiated. The bill? More than $100,000. Medicare

There truly is something wrong with our health care system, starting with the apparent fact that bills have no grounding in reality. If it costs more than $100,000 to deliver a treatment and insurance pays only a fraction of that, obviously the facility cannot keep providing the service at a loss. Yet they do. So it must not really cost $100,000 in the first place. What does it cost? No one can ever answer this question.

It seemed that the only thing that didn't "cost" anything was the time of the patient, so no one really worries too much about wasting that.

paid a fraction of that, and the rest of the bill went away.

After five treatments with Cyberknife, my life settled down into a comfortable regime of seeing the oncologist occasionally and finally being able to make future plans.

BACK TO SEA LEVEL

Since my three-month follow-up CT scan in April 2009 had produced a result of "nothing new," we decided to try, yet again, to take a vacation. We headed toward sunnier weather in Florida and a cruise on the inland waterway up the lower East Coast.

In early May, we left for Florida. Check-in for the flight from Denver to Tampa brought up the same surliness I had felt when I gave up my "priority" status with United years before, at which time I swore I'd never fly with them again. Alas, limited direct flight options to Tampa meant there was little choice this time, and so United it was.

Because I had ordered oxygen in advance for the flight, we were unable to check in online. My flight record also noted that I had requested a wheelchair so as to conserve the batteries in the portable oxygen concentrator (POC) I was carrying with me. No wheelchair was waiting for me outside at the sidewalk check-in. A United agent told us to go inside to the counter, which was quite a long walk. By the time we got there, the concentrator batteries were showing some depletion. I said to the agent behind the counter, "I really do need a wheelchair, and I need it now."

Here comes the surly part:

She: Well, you have to tell us you want it.

Me: You are the third person I have told.

She: Here? Today?

Me: Yes.

She: Who?

At this point the wheelchair showed up and I no longer had to continue wasting my breath and battery power on that conversation.

The advantage to the eventual arrival of the wheelchair was a free pass to the front of the security line, where they satisfied themselves that Roger and I weren't carrying hazardous materials. At the gate, we got early boarding. A mechanic showed up to install an oxygen tank in the overhead bin above me and to get me

When you fly with a portable oxygen concentrator, do everything you can to go onboard with totally full batteries. Airlines require that you have 1.5 times as much battery power as the length of the flight. More is better. You can top up your batteries at the gate if you arrive early enough. Better yet, stay on bottled oxygen until you board. This can be done two ways. One is to make arrangements with your oxygen company to pick up the tank at the gate after you take off. (This option probably involves a fee.) The other way is to arrange for a friend or caregiver to go the airport with you, get a companion pass from your airline to accompany you to the gate, and carry out the oxygen tank after you have embarked.

connected up to it. This effectively took up the entire over-head bin above us, and we used another bin for our carry-ons. Needless to say, we didn't make any friends when the rest of the passengers began to board, looking for places to store their own carry-ons.

After a week progressing by car from Tampa to Jack-sonville with various intermediate stops, we met Boulder friends for the week-long cruise on the intercoastal water-way. After that, we enjoyed some sunny beach time on the Isle of Palms in South Carolina before we headed home. All in all, twenty-three wonderful days near sea level, where the air was oxygen-rich compared to Colorado alti-tudes. Not needing to cart oxygen around was a blessing.

My life was little impacted by cancer in 2009. So little impacted that I actually finished my second mystery novel, *See How They Shine*. It was published March 19, 2009. I was doing so well, we even decided to join friends on their annual trek to Mexico, scheduled for January 2010.

MEXICO TRIP DERAILED

I should have known better. Our trip to Mexico was derailed by a presumed ulcer. "Presumed" meant that I had spent a lot of time over the course of several weeks trying to get a diagnosis for the sudden stomach pain that showed up four days before we were scheduled to leave for Mazatlan. Two weeks later, there were still "various possibilities" for the cause of the pain. A biopsy of stomach polyps was benign. A CT scan offered very little new information compared to the scan from ten months before. That previous scan was a treatment follow-up to determine whether the chemo and radiation had worked on the lung cancer and mesothelioma.

The initial diagnosis was that the pain was the result of scar tissue either from the surgery at Columbia-Presbyterian when the left lower lobe of my lung was removed, or—more likely in my opinion—from the empyema that had formed near where the catheters had been inserted to pour chemo directly on the meso lesions on my chest wall. Further, the idea that it was scar tissue pain seemed unlikely to me, since when I took my ulcer medication—medication that coats the inside of my stomach—the pain subsided. How could coating the inside of the stomach affect scar tissue outside the stomach?

Another result of the most recent CT scan was that now a bunch of "tiny nodules" in my right lung were more prominent than they had been on the CT scan of ten months ago. Was it lung cancer? Probably not, because the nodules had changed very little over a long period of time. Maybe inflammation from cruddy air? Maybe oxygen damage? (This was something new to ponder, that oxygen could cause fibrosis or damage to the lungs.) There was increased scar tissue in the area where the radiation was targeted and the area of the lobectomy, where Dr. Sitarik had thought the pain was originating. It was becoming more and more difficult to pinpoint exactly what was going on.

TACHYCARDIA AND THE EMERGENCY ROOM, AGAIN

A few weeks later, in March 2010, I seemed to be feeling better and getting things done—until I wasn't. During a casual lunch with friends, my heart flipped into a violent episode of tachycardia. By a violent episode of tachycardia, I mean that my heart was beating so hard I had trouble talking. I had experienced issues with a rapid heartbeat before, but this was not just a rapid heartbeat, it was heavy pounding. New and very scary.

A hurried trip to my cardiologist landed me directly in the ER. My heart eventually calmed down after several hours, but that didn't mean I got to go home. First, there was another CT scan to check for blood clots. There were none. The final diagnosis: tachycardia of unknown origin. Pretty much how all of my medical issues have been diagnosed for far too long—of unknown origin.

Annoyed by hearing yet another of-unknown-origin diagnosis, I set out on a literature search. An abstract from the journal *Cancer* reported that the results of electrocardiograms (EKGs) are abnormal in almost 90% of people with mesothelioma. A rather old journal paper reported that sinus tachycardia is the single most common arrhythmia due to tumor "invasion" of the heart. None of my doctors seemed to know about that. Curious.

In response to my constant kvetching about "unknown origins," I was sent home with a heart monitor that used Bluetooth technology for real-time monitoring of the minute-by-minute activity of my heart. I was to wear it for two weeks and keep a dedicated cell phone within ten feet of the monitor. Said cell phone recorded any cardiac "events" and I also could record them on the phone myself. I had to squeeze the phone to bring up a menu, which, of course, I couldn't read without a magnifying glass. I could then scroll down to select any symptoms I might be having along with the tachycardia. I could select from quite an array of symptoms, none of which I had experienced. I took this as a good sign. Further, I didn't experience tachycardia again during the two weeks I wore the monitor.

"STABLE DISEASE"

By the end of July 2010, I had passed yet another CT scan. The official result remained "stable disease," which meant I still had some funny-looking spots in my lung or on my chest wall (no one was really sure which), but they were the same funny-looking spots that had been there before. I have had the spot in my right lung since at least 1998, but the radiologists remained interested in it. I figured that anything that hadn't changed in twelve years was really the least of my present worries. It was probably a bean I inhaled when last I stuck beans up my nose, perhaps in 1945 or so.

There was likely only one spot that mattered: a nodule in my left lung that was there before the lung surgery in New York in October 2008. But since Columbia-Presbyterian had lost almost all of the pathology samples that the surgeon had removed during surgery before they ever got to the lab, no one knew what it was that seemed to have remained behind. Whatever it was, it hadn't changed in almost two years.

In my increasingly self-educated opinion, I thought the nodule was probably on my diaphragm and not in my lung at all. I based this estimation on two things: (1) During the original VATS in August 2007, they were going after a lung nodule that turned out to be on my diaphragm. It was also the largest of the mesothelioma lesions. They did not attempt to remove it at that time. (2) More than a year later, the surgeon at Columbia-Presbyterian did attempt to remove it but did not get clear margins. This was one of only two path samples that *did* make it to the lab. My opinion was that, in all likelihood, this "left lung" lesion was actually the meso lesion on the diaphragm.

Given the continuing stability of my disease, Dr. Sitarik decided I could wait six months instead of three to get my next CT scan. It felt like progress and tempting the fates at the same time.

Also about this time, I "graduated" from pulmonary rehab. This meant Medicare had decided that I was as good as I was going to get and thus I would no longer benefit from further supervised rehab. It wasn't a gold watch, but I did get a T-shirt and a water bottle, both cheerfully emblazoned with BCH Rehab. I still needed supplemental oxygen to do anything substantial, but I could manage around the house without it most days.

I continued to try to have a life. I found I could go to the Central City Opera (more than 9,000 feet above sea level) if someone dropped me off in front of the theater. What I should have thought of, though, was that I should have been picked up there after the opera also. Several hundred steps separated the Opera House from the parking lot. It was only slightly uphill, but even on maximum oxygen, I was gasping for breath most of the way. Seeing the opera was completely worth it, though.

TROUBLE IN PANCREAS

In the meantime, my gastrointestinal (GI) issues and stomach pain continued, but finally there was a glimpse of what might be wrong: my pancreas. Mixed in with the über-technical jargon given to me by one GI doctor was the following simple statement: "Your pancreas got old and quit." *Thanks for the commentary*, I thought. The main job the pancreas has in the body is to help break down food so it can be digested and to help regulate blood sugar levels. Mine wasn't doing either.

Besides the pain I'd been experiencing, the net result of a nonfunctioning pancreas made eating a bit of a nightmare, as my body struggled to properly digest common everyday foods. Sudden, unpredictable bouts of diarrhea intermixed with constipation were starting to substantially interfere with my life.

Now a lesson in ingenuity: two nurse practitioners put their heads together and came up with a "prescription" of sorts to mimic pancreatic enzymes and to assist with my digestion. My instant digestive symptom fix: eat, take the enzyme and digest food without incident. Sounds so simple, but that simple fix took eight weeks to get figured out. This was not the whole problem, however. Massive blood sugar swings and unreliable control of blood-thinning medications presented the next round of challenges.

ANOTHER OPERA TRIP

Attending the opera in San Francisco at sea level seemed a far better idea than trying the opera in Central City again. I set out for San Francisco with new diabetic drugs to help control the blood sugar swings. I met a friend there, and we had scheduled three nights in a row at the opera. This was my first trip without Roger since I'd been suffering the effects of cancer treatment. It was a much needed break for both of us, and we were equally excited about the idea of my achieving at least a minimal degree of independence. My pancreas, tamed for the present time by regular application of drugs, behaved for the most part, although a last-night excursion into unwise eating was—in a word—unwise. The resulting GI upset kept me in the bathroom most of the night.

Flying had ceased to be an easy task for me, each trip seeming to bring a new set of obstacles to conquer. On the way home from San Francisco, TSA somehow lost my boarding pass during the process of dumping the contents of my purse, wanding me because my metal knees set off the alarms, and testing my portable oxygen concentrator for suspect explosives. Replacing the boarding pass wasn't exactly straightforward and required me to keep my mouth shut each time "She lost her boarding pass" was uttered. *I* didn't lose my boarding pass--*they* lost my boarding pass. *Grrr.*

YELLOW EYEBALLS

Upon my return from San Francisco, I embarked on a tour of local endocrinologists, hoping to resolve the "old pancreas that quit" issue. That quickly escalated from being just a medical puzzlement to an outright emergency when I turned yellow. A CT scan on October 13, 2010, revealed a 2.5-cm mass in my pancreas. The mass was blocking the bile duct, causing bile to back up in my body, and turning my skin and the whites of my eyes a dramatic shade of yellow.

An unsuccessful attempt by a gastroenterologist to open the duct did at least yield a sufficient biopsy sample. A second try at opening the duct also failed, and so the plan shifted to inserting a stent into the blocked bile duct in hopes of clearing the blockage and draining it. An inserted stent is not 100% successful, but is much less risky than the alternative of reaming out the bile duct from the liver side. In the meantime, I was all set for Halloween with my bright yellow eyes and matching skin tone.

The two failed attempts to open and drain the blockage of my bile duct involved more than seven hours of anesthesia and a lot of IV fluids, which kicked me into congestive heart failure once again. Hence, my transfer from Foothills Hospital across town to the cardiac unit at the main Boulder Community Hospital, where they had a telemetry bed and could watch my heart closely while I awaited yet another procedure to open the blocked duct.

The third attempt worked. The stent was in and doing its job. I was, however, not out of the woods. As it turned out, the surgeon had placed a bypass catheter, not a stent, through the bile duct. This catheter emptied into my duodenum, and a collection bag was attached outside my body. Once this had been accomplished, more than a liter of thick, greenish-black bile successfully drained out of me and into the bag.

This meant that now I had a stopcock in my side. Open one side, you got bile. Open the other side to flush it out.

Flushing out the stent was to be a daily job. Unpleasant, but probably not permanent.

I was able to return home a week before Halloween and, with the help of friends, Roger was finally able to get some much-needed rest. Home Health Care started and proved to be a huge help in our day-to-day lives.

THE RESULTS OF THE BIOPSY

The pathology from the latest biopsy was unclear. The report said that the mass in my pancreas was cancer for sure. But what kind of cancer was it? Was it a new, primary pancreatic cancer? A metastasis of something else? If something else, was it one of my three primaries? Or a new one "of unknown origin"? Testing the cells, not the tissue, made it more difficult to determine what treatment, if any, would be useful.

Four days after I came home from the hospital, my liver functions started to rise (bad); some had doubled since I left the hospital and they were already high while I was there. My level of bilirubin, the stuff that made me yellow, was only slightly up, and maybe not significantly. My liver clearly did not like having a big loop of catheter in it. Would it adjust? It hadn't so far, but maybe it was still trying.

The end result of all of this hullaballoo was extreme, overwhelming fatigue and a not quite bleeding but nonetheless bloody catheter and stopcock in my side.

Between Home Health Care and an additional caregiver, I now had much-needed round-the-clock care for the foreseeable future.

A few days later, however, I was readmitted to Boulder Community Hospital for pain control. My hemoglobin level, which had been an almost healthy 12 when the turning yellow saga first began a few weeks before, tanked to 8. The overwhelming pain seemed to be coming from the catheter, so they tried to clean it out. When that didn't work, they took the catheter out and started over. The result was a *second* catheter in my liver draining bile to the outside.

We were still in limbo waiting for a possible second opinion on my "iffy" pathology report, and I had not yet had a PET scan. In short, we were right where we'd started a few weeks before. Something was clearly going on with my pancreas and liver, yet no one could tell me what.

The one thing I had working in my favor was the oncologist who was on call at the hospital that week. He was hearing my story with a fresh set of ears. I was able to talk to him about what had been going on—or had *not* been going on, as it were. He agreed with me that I had no information, that I needed more information, and that RMCC should help me get more information. To start with, he ordered a number of blood tests, looking for various cancer markers. He arranged a PET scan for the next week and sent an email to Dr. Sitarik, my regular oncologist, from his handy Blackberry while he was in my hospital room.

He also ordered a blood transfusion as well as a chest X ray, since there were crackles in my right lung. His reasoning: instead of waiting to see whether my low hemoglobin or the lung crackles would correct themselves, to just correct them and get me healthy enough to get out of the hospital and back onto my main task of figuring out where to go from there.

The immediate problem for the moment was the second stent in my liver, as this time it was gummed up and wouldn't drain properly. So it was back to the hospital to insert a permanent metal stent in my liver. This "permanent" stent was supposed to stay in good working order for at least six months. Thank goodness the surgery was successful, and a day later I was back home with Home Health Care again.

But the obvious remaining problem from the ongoing bile duct issue was that my hemoglobin was low and getting lower. Usually, this meant there was internal bleeding, but no one could actually find anything that was bleeding. Swell. My primary care doctor, Lila Rosenthal, said, "Remember, we have just begun to fight." I thought, *Maybe you have just begun, I've been doing it for perhaps too long.*

As always, my first thought was to get an opinion from MD Anderson. To that end, I had tried from my hospital room to get an appointment at MDACC and to get the pathology slides from Boulder sent to Houston. Apparently, it takes a village to collect biopsy slides, but thankfully I had a village working on my side. After many, many repetitious phone calls, emails, and back-and-forth communication, the slides were all finally assembled in one place in MD Anderson's pathology department.

Dr. Fossella, the thoracic doctor I had seen at MDACC in 2007, wanted to know which service I wanted to see when I came to Houston, a trip scheduled for January 2011. I had some choices: GI oncology, GI surgery, or thoracic oncology. *But how the heck should I know?* This was a red flag I overlooked. I should have wondered why such questions were apparently a matter of opinion, and my opinion at that.

I chose gastrointestinal oncology, and appointments were made for early January.

CHAPTER SIX

A FOURTH PRIMARY

On Tuesday, November 16, 2010, Dr. Sitarik reported that all of the medical minds had come to agree that I had pancreatic cancer—my fourth primary cancer. The first was breast cancer thirty years before, and now three more in three years. At this point, I really had to ask, *How is this possible?* The tumor was small and therefore operable, but no one thought I would survive a Whipple surgery, the only possible cure.

In general, Whipple surgery removes the tumor from the pancreas, may remove the entire pancreas, and removes, rebuilds, and reroutes most of the rest of the digestive system. In experienced hands, Whipple surgery has a mortality rate (from the surgery) of around 2%. After the surgery, however, 47% of people have serious complications while still recovering in the hospital. Notwithstanding all of that, recovery is extremely difficult and can take more than six months.

So, we were on course to first look at the most immediate issues of reducing nausea and pain. But time waits for no woman. I started chemo with Gemzar two days later. If it did not work in six weeks, it was to be Hospice time. At the suggestion of the hospital chaplain, Roger and I had a lengthy consult about Palliative Care. In the colloquial, I was not yet "circling the drain." I also didn't think I was ready for Palliative Care again yet, but maybe soon.

Thanksgiving Day was busy. We had chateaubriand from Omaha Steaks. How's that for lazy? It was delicious and we then froze five packages of it to carry along for lunch/snacks on chemo days, since the Cancer Center offered lots of food, but all of it salty, sugary, or carbs. The evening of my second chemo, this had culminated in a blood sugar of 475. Our instructions were to go to the ER if blood sugar was 500, but since I was *not* going to the ER again, I instead gave myself a huge whack of insulin, which made me jittery and sobby all night. (Ergo, no more Cancer Center snacks.)

The day I was scheduled to have my third of the six chemo treatments, I flunked the "prelims." My platelets were at a sufficiently low level that I would not receive my regular dose of chemo that day. After some discussion, Dr. Sitarik decided on a reduced dose of the Gemzar. Interestingly, my oxygen-carrying red blood cells and the infection-fighting white cells were okay; only my platelets were in the tank.

By the first week in December 2010, we were at a decision-making point. My choices were to either take a break from the chemo, which *was* working, or go on for the entire six straight weeks. According to the literature, six chemo treatments in a row were better because Gemzar apparently works best if you keep at it. Seemed like a no-brainer. The doctors, however, thought that my bone marrow wouldn't hold up for six weeks of treatment. But, since I was holding my own, the decision was made to push on.

My sixth Gemzar dose was scheduled for two days before Christmas. For the time being, it was my last scheduled Gemzar. My platelet counts were normal after this round, thanks to the reduced dosage of the chemo I'd been receiving since my platelets tanked in round three. I hoped that the reduced amount of chemo in my body was not the reason I'd been feeling better. In my exhausted mind, I preferred to think it was because the chemo was working. It was time to get an opinion from MDACC.

BEING PREPARED WHILE FLYING

We flew into Houston on New Year's Day 2011 in the hopes of experiencing less hassle than if

> If you need more than 4 lpm (liters per minute) of oxygen, you cannot fly. You also do not qualify for Angel Flight, the service that matches patients traveling for treatment with empty seats on corporate aircraft.
>
> If you do qualify, Angel Flight is worth checking out at

In the past, some airlines would provide oxygen for a price. That has stopped. It is possible to work something out with them, however, if you need to take a transoceanic flight. Follow these guidelines:

1. Start negotiations early.

2. Keep a record of everyone you talk to.

3. Try to get an email from the airline that puts any agreement in black and white.

If you have to change planes, you have a problem. Try to have a long enough connection to top up your batteries on the ground. Having a friend (or a friendly oxygen company) meet your plane with bottled oxygen lets you use that while recharging your POC as quickly as possible.

we flew on any of the other days of that holiday weekend. I had taken the time to research and print out information from the TSA website (TSA.gov) regarding passengers with hidden disabilities, and I highlighted the relevant items for my trip. Some of my disabilities are not so "hidden," but the diabetes that came with the pancreas tumor is. TSA allowed me to carry on my water bottle, two bottles of Glucerna, and a bunch of needles. Furthermore, I did not have to take off my shoes. The TSA website clearly says disabled people do not have to remove their shoes, but I had to show that sentence to the supervisor before they reluctantly agreed to it.

Instead, they swiped both my hands and my shoes with something meant to detect explosives. Another screener stuck a test strip in my water, took a squirt from the portable oxygen concentrator also to test for explosives, and did an in-chair pat down. Being prepared for all this meant that getting there was not as much of a hassle.

MDACC APPOINTMENTS

Tuesday, January 4, 2011, was my first day of appointments at MDACC, beginning early and ending very late. After this very long day of tests, the GI doctors met to decide what, if anything, they could suggest as a course of treatment for the pancreatic cancer. The decision came the next day. The Whipple surgery was not an option. Their reasoning was "concerning changes" in my chest and a newly discovered and very large lymph node in my pancreas. But what they were calling a lymph node might not actually have been a lymph node. Because it had a low density on the scan, it could be a cyst or encapsulated fluid leakage from one of the three unsuccessful attempts to put a stent in to drain my bile. A low-density "anomaly of unknown origin" was the medical-speak for this.

On the subject of surgery, the doctor at MDACC said more than 70% of people who have the horrific Whipple surgery at their institution still have recurrent pancreatic cancer. Said another way, 30% are fine. This number, 30%, is higher than most institutions produce, probably because MDACC does not operate on "iffy" people.

I knew I was "iffy," and they confirmed it. MDACC asked me to schedule my next consult for late March. We did, but headed home discouraged.

CYCLE TWO OF GEMZAR

I thought I was into cycle three of Gemzar, until I found out what "cycle" really meant. Cycle one was the six treatments I'd had in November and December. Cycle two was the three weeks on and one week off scheduled for January 2011. I had misunderstood the numbering system, which meant that I wasn't even close to being done with chemo if I had to have four cycles, and I had just finished only the second.

The preliminary test results in the third week of January were not good. Platelet levels were so low that, once again, they could give me only a half dose of chemo. Hemoglobin and other white and red blood cell measures were low. *Way* low in the case of the hemoglobin. Not yet at transfusion levels, but if the curve stayed the way it had been going, I would get there fast. Low white blood cell count meant I was suddenly more vulnerable to infection.

In addition, my liver enzymes were all whacked out. This could have been the chemo or something happening in my liver, an "early warning" on stent failure, or who knew what. I certainly couldn't think of anything good that it could be.

I also was waiting for the results of my bilirubin levels. If my bilirubin was up, it would be time to revisit the GI doctor. Likewise, I still hadn't received any word on the CA 19-9, the pancreatic cancer marker. These results could take anywhere from one day to more than one week. I was in limbo-land. Again.

But Dr. Sitarik wasn't worried. He said something to the effect of, "That's why we give you a week off, because chemo does this sort of thing." Yes, I know that, but it had not done it *all at once* before. Nor did it do it when I had six chemos in a row in November and December. Maybe I was expecting miracles.

THE DECISION FOR PALLIATIVE CARE

In late January 2011, I finally succumbed to the prodding of many friends and joined Palliative Care. This gave Roger and me access to the services of a Palliative Care team. This team included a social worker to take over "arguing" with Medicare about such things as whether I needed a wheelchair—arguments that totally wore me out and

> The goal of Palliative Care is to relieve suffering. It consists of a team effort meant to address not only the physical pain of chronic disease, but the emotional, spiritual, and family concerns that arise with advanced illness. Palliative Care is not to be confused with Hospice, which comes with the "six months to live" caveat.

usually resulted in my putting it off for too long or just giving up entirely.

There was also a registered nurse (RN), who sorted drugs, including those I was using and those I still had "just in case." The just-in-case drugs included narcotic pain meds that the Palliative Care nurse recorded as "in the house," so should we call in the middle of the night with a pain emergency, they could look up my file and, in the midst of possible chaos, quickly see whether there was anything readily available to use. The RN also came once a week to check me out and report to my oncologist and primary care doctor. She worked closely with my endocrinologist to come up with a plan to see whether we could at least quasi-control my blood sugar on chemo day and the day or so after.

Palliative Care also assigned a CNA to me. She helped with things such as showering and getting dressed. This worked for early Sunday mornings, when I wanted to go to church. Since someone had to help me shower and get dressed, previously this had meant having a caregiver show up by 8:00 a.m., when they usually started at 11:00. And even though long-term care insurance paid for eight hours a day, if the caregivers started at 8:00 (assuming one would even be willing to change her schedule for just Sunday), she would be leaving at 3:00 instead of 6:00. Then Rog would have to deal with dinner totally by himself. This resulted in my missing church most Sundays. Having the CNA help me get ready for church and let the caregivers keep their 11–6 schedule seemed a good choice. Lastly, there was a very upbeat chaplain, who visited twice monthly whether I needed her or not. Fortunately, my own pastor was also very good about staying in touch.

At this point I also signed an all-inclusive "Do Not Resuscitate" order should something happen, such as a stroke, heart attack, or a replay of the blocked bile duct. At the time, I was ambivalent about this, but it was clear that Roger and I needed help such that we wouldn't have to orchestrate on-the-spot decisions *if* they became necessary. The downside of accepting Palliative Care was that I had to agree to be "homebound." That is, I was severely limited in where I could go outside the house. In exchange for this concession, Palliative Care came to me with anything I needed, including the promise of wonderful support for both of us.

I was hoping to see a few concerts and maybe an opera or two, so I explored with the Palliative Care admissions nurse in great detail the meaning of "homebound." We agreed that I could "probably" go somewhere once a month, as long as it entailed a huge effort to get there, thus justifying my need for the Palliative Care program.

On another front, I got my official marijuana registry card so I could go to a medical pot shop but only with my designated caregiver, Roger, who had the only legal copy of my registry card. Given that Colorado endorsed medical pot, they certainly made it difficult to get in the loop. Both I and my physician had to fill out all the forms twice because I did something wrong on the forms the first time. (And they had to be notarized. *Grrr.*)

The State of Colorado cashed my check and then sent the forms back pointing out my error and giving me three weeks to respond by doing the forms over or losing my deposit and having to start the process over again.

I had hopes that pot would address both the pain and nausea issues, which at that time seemed to be mostly nonissues. But the occasional episodes of both were probably harbingers of things to come, so I thought it best to be ready.

EXISTENTIAL THOUGHT

Throughout January, I had received a mountain of emails from friends and family, all wanting to know how I was feeling about everything that was happening. I gave the same response to everyone by email, hoping to cover all of my bases in one shot.

> *I am bummed out. I still hope that Gemzar will keep working, but have less confidence that it will. I find it harder and harder to do anything, which could be the low hemoglobin, or it could be general despair hovering in the near foreground.*

> *I'm better than I used to be because I'm not on narcotics. But the narcotics were battling the stent pain issues, not the cancer.*

I'm worse than I used to be because my blood sugar issues really distress me, both mentally and I think physically.

Friends are taking up some of the slack in meal prep, but it is almost impossible to tell anyone what I can eat day-to-day. So it is depressing when people want to help and I have to keep saying no that won't work, or whatever.

I would say I feel scared, annoyed, and grateful for having so many friends!

I also feel an increasing urgency to "decide" what to do about further treatment, about returning to MD Anderson in early April, as they want me to do, about monitoring the stent (which apparently cannot really be done), about seeing if anyone besides me cares about what is going on in my left lung. I guess those are the big decisions pending.

The overarching issue of all of the above decisions was my usual need to be in control. That was becoming less and less possible. Just as an example: one of the times when they had me all hooked up to the steroid and were ready to start the Gemzar, I remembered to say, "You know I'm only getting a half dose today, right?" The response was a puzzled "Really?" and an exit to "go check." So I got the half dose. They did check everything twice, but the half-dose decision was made only 15 or 20 minutes before I got to the chemo room, and the drugs were usually pre-mixed before that. I remembered to mention it only moments before the bag of chemo would have been connected to the IV already running. Soon, I feared, I wouldn't be remembering things, and that was scary in a different way.

DECIDING THE NEXT COURSE OF TREATMENT

The day after my next full chemo treatment in February 2011 (cycle three), I felt pretty good, and the blood tests came out "great." My hemoglobin count went up from 10.2 to 11.8. Normal at this altitude is 12.6–16.3. Mine wasn't normal, but it was a darn sight better than it had been. The most amazing result to me was the platelets count, which had been down to a very low 71,000, but had come back up to 339,000 after the chemo (normal is 174,000 to 412,000). My white blood cell count was back into normal range. The white blood cells are the ones that help to fight infection, so being "back to normal" meant I would be able to go to church without worries.

If I wound up having radiation, then the next decision would be whether to do it concurrently with chemo (called "radio-sensitizing"), which would make the radiation work better. If the answer was yes to chemo, then the question involved which drug.

So the decision was complicated and multifaceted. Who would make this decision? Either the tumor board at Boulder Community Hospital, which included oncologists, radiation oncologists, interested other doctors, therapists, and the like, or the group at MD Anderson. Was there a vote? I don't know. Who had a voice? Everybody. Who had the loudest vote? I thought it likely that Medicare guidelines and a desire on the part of the doctors to not be liable for malpractice, at the very least, got the *last* vote.

I had initially planned to go back to MD Anderson in late March or early April and skip the decision part at Boulder Community altogether. But with the way the cycles were "numbered," there was almost a month between the end of cycle three and my next scheduled appointments in Houston. Added to that was the fact that BCH wanted me to have cycle four completed before I went to Houston, which MD Anderson did *not* want me to do.

In short, I was becoming concerned about the course of my treatment. Everything I had read or been told seemed to indicate that keeping up the pressure on the tumor was a good thing. In other words, if the chemo was working, don't stop. If you stop, it might give cells that were just staggered and not killed by the chemo the ability to regain their strength. To wait a month could be a problem.

So what to do?

I sent an email to my doctor's assistant at MD Anderson saying I seemed to have a lot of choices: go without treatment for more than a month, go with treatment recommendations at RMCC and preclude any input from MDACC, or go to MDACC in early March. Noting that only one of these options seemed wise to me, I asked whether they agreed. I guess they did because I suddenly had appointments scheduled in Houston for early March. For the record, I had twice before asked for appointments in early March, and both times I was told, "No, do another cycle of Gemzar and then come in April."

This would likely be my last trip to Houston. Flying was now a major hassle and, as it turned out, not worth it. They turned me down again for surgery at MDACC.

TACHYCARDIA YET AGAIN

After my last episode of tachycardia in 2009, I had gone to see my cardiologist, who sent me immediately to the emergency room. And, again, to the ICU. When he discharged me several days later, he told me, "Go to the ER if this happens again and if it worries you." I remember querying him on the instruction "if it worries you," and getting only a repeat, "if it worries you."

So when my heart rate jumped to 140 in late February 2011, I decided not to worry about it. I did not call the triage nurse at Palliative Care, as I was supposed to do if there was a problem, because I knew there was likely nothing she could do except send me to the ER, and I had had enough of ERs. Nor did I call anyone else for the same reason.

Dr. Sitarik once said at an earlier meeting, "Doing the same thing and expecting a different result shouldn't be anything we try after we've gotten out of kindergarten." I agreed. I had gone the ER/ICU route twice with tachycardia—once too often, since I had been out of kindergarten a very long time.

The tachycardia lasted all weekend. By Monday morning, I was exhausted and debating whether there was maybe a limit to how long a seventy-two-year-old heart can beat that hard. I didn't think I had a blood clot and, as I was already on daily blood-thinning shots for the pancreatic cancer, I didn't think the ER would do anything that I wasn't already doing, except maybe stick me in the ICU again and cause a lot of worry to me and those around me.

That day, my caregiver took me to a scheduled acupuncture appointment at Integrative Care at Rocky Mountain Cancer Center. The acupuncturist noted my heart rate, commented on it, and made me promise to go upstairs to see the RMCC triage nurse after my acupuncture appointment.

Shortly before noon, she went upstairs with me. I checked in at the triage desk and started the whole thing off by insisting that I was *not* going to the ER. Period. The nurse checked with a doctor and they decided that maybe it was just anemia, so we began a round of blood tests. The results: not anemic. I still refused to go the ER. Finally, we negotiated an agreement: I would get an EKG, and if anything looked strange, I would go to the ER.

Thus began the day's lesson: be careful what you agree to, even on your own terms. It turned out I couldn't get the EKG at the Foothills Hospital campus, where RMCC is located, but instead had to go across town to BCH. By this time, it was well past lunchtime and my newly diabetic persona was feeling crabby. Of course, my caregiver and I had only a 12-carb snack with us, no test equipment, and no insulin. Hence, we went home to collect the diabetic supplies and to tell Roger what was going on. I had left the house a few hours before "just to go to an acupuncture appointment." *No big deal* was my thought when I left that morning.

But that "no big deal" was getting bigger by the minute. I had been going with the flow all day as the situation escalated, but Roger got hit with it in one fell swoop. He was much more worried than I was when I told him what was going on. After I left, he spoke with a friend from church, who quickly sent out an email to our prayer chain. Roger, the church friend, and countless others were getting increasingly worried while I was at Taco Bell having lunch before going to the hospital for the EKG. (Yes, one regular crunchy taco has only 12 carbs.)

When we got to BCH, it turned out they had been waiting for me, worried about where we had been for "so long." I told them, "Getting my blood sugar equipment." I left out the part about Taco Bell. I barely had time to sit down before they called me back for the EKG. Guess what? It showed a fast, but extremely regular sinusoidal rhythm. So back home I went, many hours after leaving for a 50-minute acupuncture appointment, with my heart still clicking along at a hugely fast rate.

At this point I was not worried, but I was distressed. After I took an Ativan for anxiety, the distress passed, but my heart rate did not slow. It was not until the next day that I found out how many people had been worried about me. I certainly appreciated everyone's concern and thanked them for their prayers. Maybe they helped keep me out of the ICU this time.

Sometime that night, my heart rate finally dropped back to around 90. This wasn't normal, but it was a whole lot better than where it had been earlier at 140. It was still elevated, but not often above 100, and it was no longer pounding hard, just beating.

Why did this happen? No one seemed to know, but there were some possibilities. High among them was a mesothelioma lesion on the pleura of my heart. The only way to know if that was truly the case was to cut me open and take a little look-see. This was not an option, given that there wasn't anything that could be done if it turned out to be true.

Regarding my fast heart rate, I asked Dr. Sitarik, "If I do have a blood clot, what would you do differently than what you are already doing?" His answer included trying (I noted that word, *trying*) a different blood thinner, surgery if the blood clot threatened life, or using the clot-busting drug Streptokinase.

> When presented with "a need for surgery" to check out the cause of a symptom, you should ask the doctor, "OK, if what you suggest turns out to be true, what would you do about it?" If the answer is "Nothing," it for sure helps you decide whether you really need the surgery.

I decided to push the issue a little further, and said, "You'd really have someone operate on me at this point?" He equivocated, big time. Then I added a true statement: "Streptokinase killed my mother in 1989. Seems I recall it's contraindicated in anyone over seventy because blood vessels might be too thin to withstand it. My blood vessels have certainly been challenged already by various chemos. And I'm certainly over 70. Streptokinase might not be a very good idea." He replied with something like, "You'd probably not be a candidate for Streptokinase."

I was, however, a candidate for some sea level air. After talking to Dr. Sitarik and Roger at length about the fact that I was happier, healthier, and more active at sea level without supplemental oxygen, we agreed that I should go back to sea level when possible.

MUCH-NEEDED TIME OFF

When possible was early April 2011. We decided to fly to Jacksonville to visit Roger's brother and enjoy a few days of sunshine and the beach before catching a tour back to St. Augustine. The only route from Denver to Jacksonville required changing planes in Nashville, and our flight schedule allowed only fifty minutes between planes. We were late, but Southwest Airlines actually held the plane and wheelchaired me to it, so I didn't have to hurry dragging the portable oxygen concentrator while using up my oxygen at a great clip. Kudos to SWA.

The trip to Florida was good. Much warmth and sun. But our return trip involved a horrible experience on a Southwest Airlines flight because of my POC. Because I am a "person of size" (a SWA euphemism for fat), I had purchased an extra seat. Now, I probably don't actually qualify for Southwest's definition of "too fat to fly" because I can put the armrests down in the seat (barely). But I am also very tall so I need to put my feet under the seat in front of me. If I put the armrests down, there is only one way I can sit in the seat, and putting the bulky POC under the seat in front of me means there is nowhere to put my feet except right in front of me with bent knees. The flight from Tampa to Denver is almost four hours, and since I've had blood clots twice, I bought the extra seat to have the extra foot room.

The flight attendant started picking on me the moment I boarded. She admonished me that I had to have the POC "against the wall" and that I had to be in the window seat. My understanding had always been that, indeed, I have to be in the window seat with the POC against the wall but only for takeoff and landing. This is to be sure that no one

Oxygen-dependent passengers are at the mercy of the airlines. If you need oxygen, you are, by definition, disabled. So rules and regulations are controlled by the Department of Transportation (DOT), not the Federal Aviation Administration. DOT decided that POCs (portable oxygen concentrators) were acceptable. After testing, DOT published a list of specific brands of POCs that were allowed on airlines; however, within the broad guidelines of DOT rules, different airlines can have very different requirements.

So the first thing you must do is check with the airline you intend to fly. At a minimum, they will have a form that you and your doctor must fill out. This form is good for only a year. Remember to keep it updated if you fly frequently.

gets tangled in my oxygen cord while trying to evacuate the plane upon an emergency. Fine, no problem.

However, at sea level in Tampa, I don't need oxygen. So I sat in the window seat and stashed the POC under the extra seat beside me. The flight attendant came completely unglued and started yelling at me that she had told me where to put it and that it wasn't there. We argued, but she apparently couldn't hear anything I was saying. She got the gate agent to come and talk to me, backed up by someone from the cockpit—probably the copilot.

Fortunately, the gate agent heard me when I said, "But I'm not using it until we get to altitude. I don't need it for takeoff here." She seemed to understand, had a brief conversation with the ominous "back-up guy" and they both left. We took off. Within ten minutes of takeoff, my oxygen saturation was down to 87% (normal saturation is 93–100%) and my heart rate had risen above 100, so I decided it was time to put the oxygen on. The flight attendant showed up and told me yet again, "You have to have it in front of you—it cannot be in front of the empty seat next to you." I pointed out that no one was going to be evacuating at 30,000 feet, and that "against the wall" only applied to takeoff and landing.

It was an FAA rule, she argued, and she couldn't change the FAA rules. She implied that I would be arrested when we reached Denver if I didn't comply with her commands. So, I sat with my feet jammed against the POC, unable to move from the one position in which I and the POC could fit into the space of one seat. I did this for four hours at significant risk of a blood clot. Further, when we arrived in Denver, I was detained at the aircraft doorway, drawn aside, and lectured by four Southwest Airlines personnel. They showed me their in-flight manual. (I had asked to see the FAA regulation that the flight attendant had so frequently cited, but instead they showed me their manual.)

Indeed, the SWA manual does say that the POC must be against the wall for takeoff and landing, which I had not questioned. It further stated that the POC has to be under the seat in front of the passenger, but this "regulation" does not address takeoff and landing. It just says "under the seat in front." In my opinion, this requirement is there to make it clear that the POC user cannot sit at the bulkhead. This "regulation" is also not correlated with purchasing an extra seat. Common sense would dictate that, at cruising altitude, one could put the POC anywhere, just as other passengers can get their carry-ons out and do whatever they like with them. But there seemed to be no common sense operating here. Instead, everyone was focused on straightening out the old lady who had caused trouble.

In the interest of starting the hour's drive from the airport to home while I still had some battery power left in the POC, I quit arguing, but I knew they were wrong and decided to prove them so. According to a quick web search, I found that there is no relevant FAA regulation because the FAA apparently abdicates all issues of disability to the Department of Transportation (DOT). There are relevant DOT regulations. I forwarded copies of the regulations and a letter explaining why they were wrong to the Chief Executive Officer of Southwest Airlines.

In response to my letter, good news came from Southwest Airlines. While not actually admitting that I was right, the letter did say that the Manager of Passenger Safety had reviewed my request and that he felt okay with my putting the oxygen concentrator anywhere I wanted during the flight. The letter further promised a clearance written on Southwest Airlines letterhead that I could carry along with me in case I needed to show it to anyone on one of their aircraft in the future. The truly amazing thing is this: Southwest Airlines refunded all four tickets: mine,

Roger's, the concentrator's, and that of the caregiver who had been traveling with us. This after I said very specifically in my letter that I was not asking for a refund, as that was not my issue. I wanted an answer I could count on. I got both.

CHAPTER SEVEN

FROM BOTH SIDES

J oni Mitchell's lyrics, "I've looked at life from both sides now," rang some bells for me at music therapy. I tried to look at my current and my future life from "both sides."

The present "side" involved proceeding on my same treatment course, which was that I was responding exceptionally well to a relatively tolerable chemotherapy. When the chemo failed, which I was assured by both my physicians and the literature that it would, I still had options. These included reducing the dose of the current chemo, changing or adding another drug to the "cocktail," adding radiation, and, as always, Hospice.

Hospice would be the end point of all other options except for the other "side," surgical removal of the tumor. Hospice becomes a good choice usually no later than nine months after the initial diagnosis of pancreatic cancer. As I had been diagnosed on October 10, 2010, I was pushing six months in April 2011.

Given the miraculous success I was having with Gemzar, it was reasonable to expect that I would make it past the median nine months, but it was not reasonable to expect that I would survive this cancer without surgical intervention, and in the meantime, the only hope I had was that I might live a little longer without exacerbating the burden of staying alive. That is, the impact my condition had not only on me, but also on the people who love and support me.

THE CASE FOR WHIPPLE SURGERY

Why did I think it was worth trying to have a Whipple? The short answer: it would give me a shot at surviving. Roger feared it would shorten my life. Should I die from the surgery, this would obviously be true. In a sense, the surgery was an "up or down" vote. If I am not one of the unfortunate 2% who die in surgery, I would have a long recovery. But the surgery and subsequent recovery would actually be moving toward the possibility of a better, and certainly longer, life. It would not be treading water with no port in sight, as I had been doing up until then. I began to explore the possibility of having Whipple surgery somewhere other than MDACC.

Because of the mesothelioma and BAC, there was no promise that any surgeon would even consider me for Whipple surgery. More than likely, I would be unable to find an institution willing to designate me a sufficiently adequate candidate for surgery. In that case, I'd be stuck right where I was. But, until then, there was no harm in looking.

Also, I had to finish the next three chemo treatments in this cycle of Gemzar. Then a subsequent CT scan would still have to support the current "no mets" finding.

Whipple surgery has a better success rate at institutions that do a lot of these surgeries. Conventional wisdom sets "a lot" at a minimum of seventy a year. So I would have to find an institution that did a lot of Whipple surgeries. More important, I would have to find one who would actually agree to operate on me.

I started to look at the possibilities. MD Anderson, which already said they would not operate on me, remained my institution of choice. I asked them to reconsider, since National Jewish believed that there was currently nothing in my lungs to preclude successful pancreatic surgery. There were other options for surgery—Johns Hopkins, University of Maryland, and the Mayo Clinic, all of whom were doing a substantial number of Whipple surgeries, some even minimally invasive.

ON TO BALTIMORE

Thus May 2011 found us traveling yet again, this time to Johns Hopkins in Baltimore. We went to consult with their Multidisciplinary Pancreatic Cancer Team about the possibility of my having surgery there. Johns Hopkins does more than 400 Whipple surgeries every year—the second most in the world. A day-long evaluation, a detailed explanation of their pancreas protocol, and a comprehensive treatment plan that may or may not include Whipple surgery, depending on their tests, opinion, and experience.

Roger and I met with each member of the Cancer Team, which included a radiation oncologist, an oncologist, a surgeon, a social worker, a nutritionist, and the program coordinator. After reviewing the CT scans and my medical records, the Cancer Team at Johns Hopkins offered me three treatment scenarios.

Option one: Continue chemo at the present dose in preparation for a twenty-five-day regimen of radiation at RMCC in Boulder. While undergoing radiation treatment, I would stay on a radio-sensitizing dose of Gemzar. This meant enough Gemzar to make the tumor more sensitive to radiation.

Option two: Immediate surgery to remove the tumor in my pancreas.

Option three: Wait a few months and see what happens.

Option one was the suggested treatment, and the one I chose. The twenty-five-day radiation treatment was scheduled to be finished around the Fourth of July. Two to three weeks of "rest" later, I would have a CT scan, which would be sent to Johns Hopkins. If everything looked okay at that point, I would return to Baltimore in August for pre-op evaluation.

THE JOHNS HOPKINS PLAN

Visiting Johns Hopkins turned out to be an empowering experience. I now had the possibility of a *curative* surgery. The bottom line was this: Johns Hopkins was willing to do the surgery if the anomalies in my lungs "behaved," if the pancreas tumor got smaller, and if the cancer didn't spread before, during, or after the radiation treatment. A lot of "ifs" in this scenario.

But it was good news. Since good news often is accompanied by not-so-good news: the 3-D CT scan taken during the "pancreas protocol" at Johns Hopkins showed the tumor starting to invade my inferior vena cava, one of the two large veins that feed blood back to the right atrium of the heart. It had not been reported before, and might not have been seen without the pancreas protocol CT scan done at Johns Hopkins. In other words, it could have been there all along, but no one knew for sure.

Cancer can be removed from a vein, but it adds time and risk to an already long and risky surgery. The tumor crowding my vein had forced my body to develop "collaterals" to help carry blood along with the affected vein. These collaterals could also potentially carry cancer cells along in my bloodstream and create a hazard for spreading the cancer.

The next thing to consider was the stent in my liver. In an ideal situation, it would continue to function for another few months and then be taken out during surgery. If it failed midway during radiation, however, that could present a problem. There was much discussion about replacing it immediately, but in the end, the final decision was something along the lines of "Let's just hope it holds up."

As to the Whipple surgery, it was estimated that I would be in the hospital for ten days, followed by at least another week "in the area" before being able to fly home. I thought that sounded most optimistic. Given that it took us eight hours to get from our Baltimore hotel to our front door in Boulder, I could not imagine handling such a trip so soon after major surgery.

I was also completely exhausted, and it was clear that I needed to work on getting my physical stamina back. I was soon to enter a new treatment regimen. I had little idea what twenty-five days of radiation coupled with daily chemo was going to do to me.

Performance status is how oncologists describe physical condition. Mine was very low, "3 going on 4" when I first got out of the hospital with the pancreatic cancer diagnosis. (Performance status 5 is dead.) Since then I had increased my performance status to 2.

NEW CHEMO AND RADIATION REGIMEN

When I began my new chemo regimen in Boulder in June 2011, it was not with Gemzar but with a new drug, Xeolda, an oral chemo pill to be taken twice a day. This was because Gemzar had apparently stopped working the end of May. My CA19-9, which had fallen from 2500 to 37, had begun going up ever so slightly since the first of April: 52, then 55, then 61, then 91. (Normal is 55 and below.)

The plan was that I would take Xeolda five days a week for five weeks along with radiation in an attempt to shrink the tumor away from my vein. That totaled twenty-five "treatments." (I put "treatments" in quotes because I believe in a few decades people will look back and wonder how we could apply such a benign word as "treatment" to the barbaric things we do today to treat cancer.)

After the chemo and radiation, the results of another CT scan would hold the deciding details. If there had been no progression of the cancer, then we would go back to Baltimore, to Johns Hopkins, and hopefully move forward with surgery to remove the cancer in my pancreas along with parts of various organs below the diaphragm. If we managed to stay on schedule, we expected to be in Baltimore in early August for surgery and home by Halloween, maybe sooner. In fact, the entire schedule had been defined by "maybe sooner, maybe later."

"Maybe never" remained a very real possibility for the next two months. For various scheduling reasons, I couldn't start radiation until June 13, which was the Monday that Verdi's *Macbeth* was to be broadcast to the Boedecker Theater in Boulder at 12:30. I therefore decided that radiation could not start until Tuesday, June 14. It was to be accompanied by Xeolda, an oral chemo pill to be taken twice a day. I proposed not doing chemo at all, just the radiation. Not a good idea, according to everyone on my cancer dance card. That included my oncologist in Boulder, the local radiation oncologist, and the doctors at Johns Hopkins.

The Xeolda pills were a problem. They were big and difficult to swallow. The oncologist had assured me that it was okay to grind them up and mix them with water. "Dissolve them in water in a paper cup, drink the water, refill the cup with water, drink that, crush the cup, staple it shut, put it in a plastic, sealable bag, and bring it to the Cancer Center for toxic waste disposal." Such instructions certainly highlight the chemo part of chemotherapy.

Radiation was very much "routine" in that I arrived, went into the waiting room, and read maybe one page of a *People* magazine before someone came to fetch me. I reserve reading *People* for when I'm in a medical waiting room. Its editorial "content" seems ideally matched to my attention span in such situations.

The actual radiation was three blasts, each at a different angle and each apparently 15 seconds long. That's according to my one-thousand-one, one-thousand-two, etc. counting. It takes more time to get me into the right position than the actual treatment takes. So, it's all fast and easy.

That is, it's all fast and easy until the machine breaks. It did so only once. The problem was a blown circuit breaker. No one could tell me why the circuit breaker failed and I rather thought that was information it would be good to have before getting back on the table for the last two blasts of radiation. However, everyone assured me that the machine wouldn't work if anything was wrong, that there are so many defaults in the machine that nothing could go wrong, etc., etc.

I argued that s**t happens and suggested I'd just go home and come back the next day. They insisted that, having had one field treated and not the other two, quitting for the day midtreatment would be a huge problem, might even compromise the whole course of treatment because it's important to have the same amount of radiation every day, every day, every day (except, of course, if there is a holiday, for example, the upcoming Fourth of July).

I didn't doubt that it might be a problem for them because someone would have to recalculate total dose and figure out how to handle one field being treated on one day and not the other two that day. However, it wasn't clear to me how it was a problem for me.

In summary, I'd had only two of twenty-five planned radiation treatments and already everyone in the place knew me as some variant of the "old lady who wanted to just go home after a circuit breaker blew."

By July 4, I was looking forward to three whole days "off" . . . no chemo pills, no radiation. Three whole days to recover. I'd had fourteen of the twenty-five planned treatments and was still seeking the primo antinausea regime. Zofran worked fairly well for six hours. You could, however, take it only every eight hours. Pot cookies/chips/candy worked very well but decidedly did *not* mix with Zofran. The day I tried both was a memorable day for me and many people at the Cancer Center. They put me on their own oxygen for the radiation scenario. So, there I was, seated on the table, playing with the cannula for their oxygen dispenser because I couldn't figure out "which way" it went on.

Then, when they were doing the treatment, I lost track of how many times the machine had moved and decided it had done so an extra time. So I told them to stop the machine. They always say, "Don't worry. We can hear you. If you have any problems, just call out."

Uh-huh. Yes, they could hear me but apparently not well. One of the techs came in: "What did you say?" I reiterated that they had already done three fields so how come they were moving the machine to set up for a fourth? She said it was a third, not a fourth. I said, "Nope, you've done three already." Upshot of all this was she swore to me that I was wrong. I decided, well, maybe I was wrong since I had no idea what was what anyway.

It turned out that was also my day to see the radiation oncologist, a once-a-week event. That conversation was "really funny," according to my caregiver who was along at that point. Mostly, I just remember that the radiation oncologist wasn't listening to me. Conclusion: Pot or Zofran. Not both! Whew!

RESEARCHING NANOKNIFE™

By July 14, 2011, I had twenty-three of the twenty-five planned chemo and radiation treatments under my belt, leaving me almost nonfunctional. As I thought my next decision might be my last chance to make any possibly meaningful choice, I'd been devoting what useful cognitive time I had to trying to get more information about a newspaper clipping a friend had sent me. It was about the use of NanoKnife technology in pancreatic cancer surgery. NanoKnife can be a minimally invasive cancer treatment that precisely targets and kills difficult-to-reach tumors. It uses a pulsed DC current to destroy tumor cells. It is not a knife.

My Internet research suggested NanoKnife might be useful to me in that it could treat a tumor next to or even surrounding a blood vessel without the need to cut into the vein. I had significant vein occlusion and possible artery involvement. This blood vessel involvement increased the already statistically lousy odds of treating pancreatic cancer. Survival rates at five years are 4%. With a successful Whipple surgery, they climb to maybe 20%. But that's 20% of the 4% eligible for surgery.

Very grim odds, with a horrific surgery the only possible shot at cure. Anything that could lessen the impact of the surgery looked good to me. An attempt at curative surgery with NanoKnife would still involve a very Whipple-like procedure, but the pancreas part of it might be greatly simplified by using NanoKnife. Simplification meant less surgery time, hence less risk.

A number of US institutions, including Baylor, Sloan-Kettering, and University of Maryland, offered Nano-Knife, but the only ones with extensive experience actually using it in the treatment of pancreatic cancer were not such big guns. Stony Brook Medical School in New York and University of Louisville in Kentucky were among the first to use NanoKnife in a Whipple procedure.

Although at the time there were no clinical trials in the United States using NanoKnife to treat pancreatic cancer, there was one recruiting in Italy. Stony Brook did the first pancreas surgery with NanoKnife in October 2010. That patient died the following February. University of Louisville had done the most pancreas surgeries with Nano-Knife, thirty-two at least.

There was also a doctor in Denver who practices at Swedish Medical Center. At that time, he had used Nano-Knife a few times, three of them in pancreas surgery. I made an appointment with him.

All that said, there was a lot of testimonial information on various cancer blogs. They seem evenly split between reports from caregivers whose patients died after Nano-Knife treatment and reports from other patients themselves who raved about how it saved their lives. I was in email contact with four folks—two each from Stony Brook and Louisville, one each of the "not so great/great" attitudes.

Obviously, getting information from fellow patients was not the ideal way to go, but there did not seem to be much else available. I did not yet have a follow-up appointment with Johns Hopkins. Essentially, they wouldn't talk to me until I got the all-important CT scan of August 2. Then, if the CT showed no mets, they would schedule an appointment for me. When? Oh, who knew? Did it matter when? Well, they said so when we were there in May. Two of them said, specifically, "The maximum response from chemo/radiation is four weeks after radiation ends. That is the best time for surgery."

I had an appointment with the University of Maryland for August 12 and with the University of Louisville for August 15. Further, the latter scheduled me for Whipple/NanoKnife surgery on August 17.

I had hoped to go to Johns Hopkins first, on August 9 or so, but that looked like an impossible goal. So, it was either bag everything else and just wait until Johns Hopkins decided whether they would see me, or go to Baltimore, see University of Maryland people, go to Louisville, see NanoKnife guy, go back to Baltimore if Johns Hopkins was willing to see me. How doable was that plan? Not very under good circumstances. And I was not in anything like good circumstances.

TRYING TO SCHEDULE NANOKNIFE SURGERY

At this point, "future planning" consisted only of the consult in early August 2011 with the surgeon at Swedish

Medical Center. This Denver option was looking better and better. The downside of the Denver option was that, of my available options at that time, Swedish Medical Center had done the fewest Whipple surgeries. Furthermore, I would start off compromised by the need for oxygen in Denver, which I did not need at sea level. The upside to surgery in Denver was that it was close to home.

I decided to back off on making a decision until the following week, when I hoped to feel better. It was clearly not a time to be making important decisions. A week later, my brain began to squish out from the ton of bricks that had fallen on it. As I understood it, radiation "damage" would continue for about two weeks after the radiation stopped. Each day was supposed to be incrementally better. I guess that was true enough.

I tried to think about NanoKnife, but my head remained in a weird disconnected place. Many facts, ideas, and thoughts, mostly unconnected to anything else, rolled randomly around in my mind. No reliable, linear thinking and really nothing that made much sense.

The newspaper was particularly puzzling. I read about a massacre that had taken place in Norway and got it confused with Oklahoma City. Somehow, the shooters looked like the same guy to me, I guess.

Often I asked Roger why a cartoon was funny. "Because it is" was his usual unsatisfactory answer. But music remained good. I watched the opera *Don Carlo*, and then spent an hour or so wondering what Spain had to do with Flanders in the sixteenth century. Seemed to me that France was between Spain and Flanders (assuming Flanders was Belgium). So why did the Spanish king oppress Flanders? Not the point of the opera? Well, it seemed to me to be exactly the point. The music was great, but *Flanders*? Did any of that really happen?

A high school friend of mine who was also a cancer survivor responded to my lament about brain malfunction. She said after radiation and chemo she was "alive but trashed." That about said it all. In her words:

> *Your description of your weird brain function reminds me so much of what I went through after treatments ended, especially the part about thoughts occurring as disconnected pieces. I had so much brain trauma that I couldn't even find the words to describe my problems, yet I knew things weren't right "up there." Finally, after two years, I tried to tell my oncologist that I was having these serious issues. She had little to offer and said that I had to expect to decline at my age, which really bugged the hell out of me!*

> *My internist, though, took me seriously and gave me a strict regimen to follow: a heavy daily dose of B-12, regular daily exercise, adequate sleep every night (which required medication because I could no longer sleep normally), and, of course, proper nutrition. It*

took one whole year on this regimen before I experienced a meager improvement.

My friend's opinion was that basically medical science, and especially the field of oncology, is very slow to acknowledge the damage cancer treatments cause or to accept any responsibility for follow-up rehabilitation. She told me about Dr. Julie Silver at Harvard Medical School, who was on a one-woman campaign to change that, and gave me some of Dr. Silver's published articles to read. Her email continued:

I began to document all of my brain issues and how long it took to see any improvements. I copied off Dr. Silver's articles, and armed with these and my brain damage-and-recovery records, I arrived for a checkup with my oncologist. I was prepared to start my own personal campaign to sell the idea of post-cancer treatment rehabilitation to her.

What surprised me was how eager she was to have my damage-and-recovery records. She explained that cancer research is done on much younger populations, and that there really aren't any good records on how the treatments affect senior patients or to what extent we recover.

My friend's words resonated with me. I too was "alive but trashed." Probably most cancer survivors are.

I attempted to talk with Dr. Sitarik about my brain dysfunction. He said I was "missing the executive function," and that some people never use theirs so they don't miss it when it's gone. He didn't think the dysfunction was brain mets, but rather a result of radiation, trauma, stress, and maybe too much Valium. I started crying. Then he sort of teared up, gave me a prescription for something other than Valium, and a big hug.

Later, when I got home, I turned to the Internet for a definition of "executive function," the part of my cognitive armada that was allegedly impaired. It turns out that it is some sort of auto-response that "initiates appropriate responses to context and inhibits inappropriate responses." It was the inappropriate responses that had been terrifying me. I knew when I was doing something totally irrational, such as crying, throwing the remote at the TV screen, asking Roger, "Am I not dying fast enough for you?" It was like standing there detached, watching myself do and say these irrational, sometimes awful things. "Terrifying" was indeed the correct word.

Terrified or not, decision time was fast approaching. The timing of the surgery was a matter of urgency because the radiation, which I had finished in mid-July, would continue to destroy the area it had targeted, and after six or eight weeks, it would be too destroyed for an operation. No stress there, right?

The Denver surgeon agreed that from the looks of my CT scan, my tumor "appeared to be resectable" (that is, operable), but he reiterated the point that I was a lousy surgical candidate. He said things like: "You could be throwing your life away" and "We may buy you a year or two more but you probably won't be cured." Also, he could not use the NanoKnife to its maximum value (blowing the tumor to bits) because of the unremovable metal stent stuck to my liver tissue. Because the Nano-Knife uses high-voltage DC current, it could not be used near metal.

After about twenty minutes of this sort of lecture, he then said that he might be able to "clean up" tumor margins around veins and arteries and that maybe he could wiggle the metal out of the stent, but he thought he wouldn't be able to get it all.

WHIPPLE SCHEDULED

The NanoKnife Whipple surgery was scheduled for Friday, August 26, 2011, at 10:30 a.m. at Swedish Medical Center in Denver. The operating room was booked for six hours. I wasn't frightened going into surgery because I knew I had an active prayer chain that literally went around the world. I knew I was going to be okay. When I came out of surgery, six-plus hours later and *not* on a ventilator, I knew I truly was blessed and that I would recover. I did not yet know, and really had not even hoped for, the great result I got. The surgeon actually managed to get clean margins everywhere using NanoKnife. Furthermore, he got rid of the metal stent. Now whatever was in me was *all* me.

I felt much better than I had expected so soon after surgery. Maybe this was because the NanoKnife eliminated a lot of the scalpel work done in a traditional Whipple; that is, my surgery was probably less complex than Whipples done without the NanoKnife.

I wasn't going to be hunky-dory in a few weeks. I was, however, getting a little better each day in the classic two steps forward, one step back sort of way.

IT'S NOT OVER YET

Less then a year later, in June 2012, a very unsettling "routine" CT scan showed a mass in the tail of my pancreas and new lesions in the right lung that could be metastases of BAC, mesothelioma, or pancreatic cancer. I had not had involvement of the right chest before, so there hadn't been any treatment directed there other than the systemic chemo, which did not work. The local treatment that *did* work, Dr. Taub's catheters in New York for the chemo infusion directly into the chest wall and later radiation, had all been on the left side.

A year after my original 2007 diagnosis of BAC and mesothelioma, the lower lobe of my left lung was removed to get rid of the BAC. Presumably it was gone. But without a biopsy, the doctors could not be certain that these new spots on the right were not BAC. One of the spots might be on the pleura and was therefore most likely mesothelioma. One appeared to be inside the lung but right at the edge, which meant it could be bridged out to the pleura, which would mean it could be mesothelioma and not BAC.

I couldn't have biopsies of my pancreas and my lung at the same time. Each was too invasive. Further, risking my "good" right lung for a biopsy seemed unwise. If there was cancer in the pancreas, then the meso would no longer be considered "life threatening," according to Dr. Sitarik. Loosely said, if there was cancer in the pancreas, it would kill me long before the mesothelioma would have its own chance to kill me.

WHAT NEXT?

Now, what was I doing about all of this?

I signed up with N-of-One, an organization in Boston that would get genetic analyses of my various tumors, research the literature, make suggestions, and try to figure out genetically what different drugs might accomplish for me.

N-of-One's preliminary report appeared to have some suggestions. My lay reading of it was that most of the suggestions were with regard to what drugs *not* to use because they wouldn't help. But better to find this out their way than by taking the drugs and then discovering they didn't work. N-of-One had some ideas on what to use as well. It appeared that the best drug I could get might be Adriamycin again. But after my 1980 successful treatment for breast cancer, I was beyond my lifetime limit on that drug. It was not an option. I say "the best drug I could get" because I was not eligible for a clinical trial (too many cancers at once, heavily pretreated with other drugs, not a clean slate, etc.), so I couldn't get any drug that wasn't released by the FDA for nonexperimental use. N-of-One continued to labor and they were ready to talk to my various physicians about their findings.

Meantime, I'm reading *Portrait of a Lady*.

About the Author

Joann Temple Dennett was a science writer for more than 50 years. A graduate of Northwestern University, she received her M.S. from the Graduate School of Journalism at Columbia University and her Ph.D. from the University of Colorado at Boulder.

Dr. Dennett worked as a science writer for a number of scientific institutions, taught at the University of Colorado, and developed and managed an English-as-a-Second-Language program for foreign visitors to the Forecast Systems Laboratory of the National Oceanic and Atmospheric Administration. She was recognized for the latter by the award of a Churchill Travelling Fellowship from the English-Speaking Union.

In 2000, she turned to fiction. Writing fiction, after a lifetime of technical and science writing, was true liberation for her.

Acknowledgments

With so many people to acknowledge, it is difficult to know where to start. Marcie Geissinger was always there to help me go wherever I wanted to go. Jerene and Bob Anderson played hour after hour of Rummikub with me. (Rummikub therapy, we called it.) Ditto Dennis and Eleanor Hubbard with their Dominoes.

Carol Keig's indefatigable cheerfulness (and great food and flowers) were always appreciated. The "many Marys"—Axe, Coberly, and Wright—and several others were willing to sit through long operas with me. Lou Holden, Karen Nelson, and Janna Vannorsdel struggled to keep things on track at home—the house, the blizzard of paperwork, the inevitable arguments with insurers.

This book would not exist without the assistance of many editorial hands. As usual, Sandy Rush saved the day. I say "as usual" because we have been working together for more than 35 years. I write something that, to my mind, is clear and concise. She follows along and edits what I wrote so that it actually *is* clear and concise. I would also like to acknowledge the help of Natasha Hubbard (content editing) and Eleanor Hubbard (concept).

Many other people touched my life—my goddess circle (aka the book club), New Women at Cairn Christian Church, and folks from the Crestmoor Drive neighborhood, past and present. I am also grateful for those friends who have been willing to share their dogs so that our home was never totally bereft of doggy vibes.

Acknowledgments

Then there are many new friends from the cancer center, fellow travelers as well as those who help to keep us on the road. Fay Elliott is prominent among the former. Truly a wonder woman, Fay's peaceful blog offers much to think about. And a special thank you to the caregivers from Safe At Home who make it possible for me to stay at home, where I want to be. They are all terrific; special kudos go to Heather Harris, who has been with us since 2010.

Many friends and family came to Boulder for most welcome visits. Dick and Sheila Plotkin, Janet Richter, Anita Dobrzelecki, Julia and Phil Williamson, Ed and Ida Hassler, Helen Brigham, and Donald and Arlene Dennett all made the trek.

There are many others willing to help, and so appreciated: Pat Weis-Taylor, Rick Hinrichs, Debby and Marty Errickson, Connie and Freddie Platt, Eleanor Crandell, Sue Nash, Karen Johnson, Jo Ann Joselyn, and Kay Lowe-Wendling. And others, who kept my spirits up with entertaining and supportive messages—Eileen Edgren, Marelynn Zipser, Joan Froede, Wendy Froede, Charlie Fellenbaum, Randi Gould, Lowell Kohlrust, Faye Muly, Karen Johnson, and Cindy Zimmerman.

I am grateful for all the love, light, prayers, and good thoughts of everyone. I am very appreciative. I think such support is a major reason I have been able to keep going long past my original prognosis in 2007 of six months to live. I thank you all. Many times over!